IN THEIR OWN WORDS

12,000 Physicians Reveal Their Thoughts on Medical Practice in America

Phillip Miller
With Louis J. Goodman, Ph.D., CAE
and Timothy B. Norbeck

Content cited in USA Today, The New York Times,
The Wall Street Journal, CNN and National Public Radio!

New York

In Their Own Words
12,000 Physicians Reveal Their Thoughts on Medical Practice in America

ISBN 978-1-60037-730-3

Library of Congress Control Number: 2009939757

MORGAN · JAMES
THE ENTREPRENEURIAL PUBLISHER

Morgan James Publishing
1225 Franklin Ave., STE 325
Garden City, NY 11530-1693
Toll Free 800-485-4943
www.MorganJamesPublishing.com

ABOUT THE AUTHORS

Phillip Miller

Phillip Miller serves as Vice President of Communications for Merritt Hawkins & Associates, the largest physician search and consulting firm in the United States and an AMN Healthcare company. AMN Healthcare is the nation's largest healthcare staffing organization. Mr. Miller has over 20 years of corporate communications and public relations experience and has been cited on healthcare staffing issues in *U.S. News & World Report, The Wall Street Journal, People, USA Today* and many other news outlets. Mr. Miller has authored numerous articles on healthcare staffing and is co-author of three books on physician staffing and supply, including *Will the Last Physician in America Please Turn Off the Lights? A Look at America's Looming Physician Shortage; Merritt Hawkins & Associates' Guide to Physician Recruiting,* and *Have Stethoscope, Will Travel: Staff Care's Guide to Locum Tenens.*

Louis J. Goodman, PhD, CAE

Louis J. Goodman is Executive Vice President and Chief Executive Officer of the Texas Medical Association. Organized in 1853, TMA is a professional membership organization comprised of more than 43,000 physicians and medical students and is the nation's largest state medical society.

Dr. Goodman is a 21-year veteran of the TMA staff and has held the position of Executive Vice President for over ten years.

Under his leadership, the TMA was recognized as "America's Best Medical Society" by *Medical Economics* magazine.

Dr. Goodman's varied healthcare experience includes an11-year tenure with the American Medical Association. Dr. Goodman holds the appointment of adjunct professor at the University of Texas Health Science Center at Houston, and serves as president of the Physicians Foundation, a group of physician and medical society leaders dedicated to enhancing the medical practice environment for physicians and patients. He is an honorary member of the AMA and past president of the American Association of Medical Society Executives and the Texas Society of Association Executives. Dr. Goodman is the 2008 recipient of the TSAE "Distinguished Executive Award."

Dr. Goodman has a masters and a doctoral degree in public policy economics from New York University and has written more than 70 articles on healthcare and medicine.

Timothy Norbeck

Tim Norbeck has held a variety of prominent positions within organized medicine over the past 40 years. From 1977 to 2006 he served as Executive Director of the Connecticut State Medical Society where he established a national reputation as an advocate for physicians and the medical profession. In 1993, the Connecticut State Medical Society awarded Mr. Norbeck an Honorary M.D. in recognition of his significant contributions to the medical profession and for his diligent advocacy on behalf of physicians and patients. Mr. Norbeck began his career in organized medicine with the American Medical Association and served as Executive Director of the Rhode Island Medical Society.

Mr. Norbeck has served in a variety of other leadership positions, culminating in the Presidency of the American Association of Medical Society Executives. Mr. Norbeck has held numerous positions on American Medical Association advisory groups and was recipient of the AMA's Medical Executive Achievement Award. He currently serves as Executive Director of the Physicians Foundation, a physician and patient advocacy organization comprised of physicians and medical society leaders.

FOREWORD

If you have any interest in what doctors think or how they feel about the practice of medicine, this is a book you should not put down until you have read it from cover to cover.

Drawing on one of the largest surveys of physicians ever undertaken in America, IN THEIR OWN WORDS *gives patients, policy makers and others a bird's eye view into the hearts and souls of today's medical men and women.*

The book asks readers to conduct an experiment – to switch places with the physician examining you and to imagine what it is like to be a doctor for a day.

It invites readers to consider why what doctors think about their profession matters to the patient's own health.

It raises a vital question in this era of healthcare reform debate – will there be enough doctors to go around and will doctors be given the latitude to actually treat the patients they see?

Most important, it lets readers sift through hundreds of comments written by physicians themselves who reveal exactly what they think about the way medicine is practiced in America today .

Part wake up call, part fact finding mission, and part remedy plan, IN THEIR OWN WORDS *makes a powerful statement about medicine today and is vital reading to anyone who has ever been a patient or who is likely to be one – and that means all of us.*

~ Richard L. Reece, M.D.
Editor-in-Chief, *Physician Practice Options*
Author, *Obama, Doctors, and Health Reform*
Blogger, www.medinnovationblog.com

Table of Contents

Table of Contents

CHAPTER ONE

DOCTOR FOR A DAY

How do physicians feel about being physicians? If asked to speak directly to patients about medical practice in America today, what would physicians say? How would they change things?

Those are the questions posed by this book -- and for the most part the answers are provided by physicians themselves, hundreds of them, in their own words.

In this chapter, however, we would like to explain why these questions matter – to patients, policy makers or to anyone concerned about the quality and availability of healthcare in the United States.

In doing so, we acknowledge that the physicians' perspective is one that is not commonly considered by most non-physicians. The reason for this seems fairly obvious. Most patients, the authors of this book included, are focused on their own concerns when they see a doctor. Uppermost in the minds of patients are two questions: what is wrong with me and what can be done about it?

The physician is there to answer those questions, in as expeditious a manner as possible. It is not the patient's duty to reflect on the physician's frame of mind or to speculate on how the physician regards the current state of the medical profession.

And yet how physicians feel about being physicians has real and important consequences for patients and for the viability of the entire healthcare delivery system.

To understand why requires an examination of who physicians are and how they are different from other kinds of professionals. It requires non-physicians to put on a white lab coat (metaphorically speaking) and be doctors for a day.

Physicians – unique and indispensable

A first step in this exercise is to consider the role that physicians play within the context of the overall healthcare system.

Though medicine has evolved technologically and in many other ways in recent years, doctors remain the indispensable providers of patient diagnosis and treatment. This is most readily apparent in an emergency. One might go weeks, months, or years without thinking of physicians in any sort of concrete or abstract way.

When serious illness or injury strikes, however, one's sole objective is to see a doctor. Not a nurse, an allied health professional or an alternative medicine practitioner. A doctor.

It is physicians, and physicians alone, who have the training and knowledge necessary to diagnosis complex diseases and to conduct complex surgical procedures. It is physicians who, with a signature, admit patients to hospitals, prescribe drugs, initiate treatments, and order tests. Very little of significance takes place in medicine today that is not ordered by, monitored by, tested by, or performed by a physician. Without physicians, so the quip goes, hospitals are just empty hotels with bad food.

Yet, as vital as they are, the presence and availability of physicians often is taken for granted. We assume that in a modern, progressive country such as the United States, physicians will be available when and where they are needed.

But that is not really the case.

Physicians are not a naturally occurring part of the healthcare landscape. They are the end product of a long, arduous and expensive education and training process. Physicians are essentially a category of scientist and must complete the highest levels of training required by virtually any profession. The path to becoming a physician includes:

- 4 years of college, with course work requiring at least one year of biology, physics with lab, general chemistry and calculus. A grade point average of 3.5 or above usually is required for medical school acceptance.
- 4 years of medical school. Continued focus on biology and anatomy, with no allowance made for poor grade performance.
- 3-5 years of hospital residency training. Medical residents generally work 80 hours a week, are directly involved in patient care and may be sued for malpractice. The average annual salary of medical residents is about $35,000.
- 1-2 years fellowship for additional advanced training in surgery or diagnosis

In all, physicians may be required to complete up to 15 years of collegiate and post collegiate education and training before they are allowed to enter into their specialties and begin earning professional incomes. Medical education and training are expensive, however. On average, physicians owe $140,000 in educational debt by the time they graduate from medical school, according to the Association of American Medical Colleges.

Though all physicians have extensive training, they differ greatly in terms of what they do. There are now over 190 different medical specialties in which physicians can obtain board certification, ranging from allergy to vascular surgery. Their duties, which may include everything from diagnosing disease to transplanting organs, carry with them a very high degree of responsibility and the stress that comes with it. Lives are literally in their hands, putting them in a position that is both uniquely powerful and uniquely vulnerable. The joy of successfully intervening in a patient's life can be exhilarating; the despair of failure can be devastating.

The bar to entering the medical profession is set very high, perhaps higher than in any other profession – and rightly so. Who would want any but the most educated, well trained, motivated, caring and talented people diagnosing or operating on their loved ones or on themselves?

Rules of the game

Physicians also are different from other professionals by virtue of the unique ground rules under which they must operate. To don a physician's lab coat and be doctor for a day requires some understanding of the peculiarities of today's medical practice environment.

This environment is largely shaped by the way in which medical services are paid for in the United States.

Medicare, the government program which pays for medical services for those 65 and older, sets physician payment rates for a wide range of services which are categorized as Diagnostic Related Groups (DRGs). An orthopedic surgeon might be reimbursed $500 by Medicare for setting a simple bone fracture, and $1,000 for setting a compound fracture. Private insurance companies often set their reimbursement rates based on what Medicare pays.

The point is that physicians rarely set their own fees. Their fees are mostly dictated to them by Medicare, Medicaid, HMOs, PPOs and other third party payers. Unlike other professionals, the money paid to physicians for their services may have little or no relation to their cost of doing business. What can be even more aggravating to physicians is that sometimes third party payers influence or dictate what they can or can't do for their patients, by declining to pay for services physicians may believe their patients need.

This is not the environment in which most other professions or businesses operate. There is no "third party" barrier between the lawyer, the accountant, the computer programmer, the plumber, or the mechanic and his or her clients. Most professionals or business people set a fee, perform a service or deliver a product, and are paid directly by the customer.

For physicians, the business model is entirely different.

Imagine a plumber who replaces a pipe for a fee set by the government or by some other third party – a fee that does not cover the cost of the new pipe the plumber has been asked to install. The plumber then submits a bill – not to his client, but to a government agency or to an insurance company. The agency or insurance company then declines to pay the bill on the grounds that they do not cover that particular service under those particular circumstances. Or perhaps they do pay the bill, but at a rate 20 percent less than the plumber's cost of doing business.

It would be no surprise if, under these conditions, plumbers began to question why they became plumbers instead of electricians or members of some other trade.

In addition, while most professionals must adhere to government or industry guidelines, they usually do not have nearly the level of regulation to deal with that doctors do. The federal tax code "only" runs to 11,000 pages, while the Medicare regulatory code by which physicians must abide is 130,000 pages long. Doctors must document just about everything they do to prove they have complied with various regulations, or risk civil and criminal penalties for fraud and malpractice. When it comes to filling out documents and forms, every day for doctors is like early April tax season for the rest of us.

Indeed, the American Hospital Association has estimated that physicians must spend one hour on paperwork for every hour they spend seeing patients.

Moreover, when doctors make a mistake in the course of their duties (or when a patient *thinks* they made a mistake) they are quite likely to be sued. Unlike most of us, they can't make an error and then come in early to the office the next day to patch things up. Instead, their professional reputations may be put on the line and, even if the suit is completely without merit, they are in for some sleepless nights.

The money myth

Any doctor for a day will quickly see that the medical profession has its challenges, but he or she may assume that these challenges will be trumped by an extravagant income.

For many physicians, this is clearly not the case. Doctors are divided into two general groups: primary care physicians and surgical/diagnostic specialists. Primary care physicians include family physicians, general internal medicine practitioners and pediatricians. Some people also consider obstetrician/gynecologists to be primary care physicians. Surgical and diagnostic specialists include general surgeons, orthopedic surgeons, cardiologists, radiologists, otolaryngologists, gastroenterologists, and other "ologists."

Primary care physicians engage in work that is mostly consultative. Under current reimbursement systems, this type of work is compensated at a lower rate than the procedures that specialists typically perform. A primary care doctor in a mature practice can expect to earn between $150,000 and $200,000 a year – a good income but not extravagant riches. Because of their lengthy training, physicians begin the earning stage of their careers many years later than most professionals and in considerably more debt. Primary care doctors in particular share the same financial concerns as most middle class people. They worry about saving for retirement and putting their kids through college.

David Watson, M.D., a family physician in Yoakum, Texas who was named the 2008 Country Doctor of the Year, expressed it this way: "I don't have a second home, or an airplane or a yacht, but I do have a lot of friends. The interaction with your patients is the most rewarding thing."

Specialist physicians typically earn more than primary care doctors and may be better off financially, though vary rarely are they in the same monetary category as successful bankers, stock brokers, entrepreneurs, corporate executives, or high powered attorneys. With few exceptions, they are not among the rich or the super-rich. Given the extent of their training and the nature of their work, which may include operating on a child's brain or transplanting a human heart, it can be argued that specialist physicians fully merit the high compensation they may receive.

As an avenue for obtaining riches, however, neither primary care nor specialty medicine hold as many possibilities for intelligent, motivated and hard working individuals as do a variety of other fields.

Where do you stand?

After spending the day as a doctor, where might you stand relative to the medical profession? What might you think about being a physician given the current state of the medical practice environment?

Suppose, after all those years of training, you felt that third parties were intervening between you and your patients, compromising your ability to provide them with the care they need -- what steps would you take? Suppose you felt that the continual fight for reimbursement and the fear of malpractice were beginning to outweigh the joy you derive from seeing patients -- what changes would you make?

Would you continue to see the same number and kind of patients? Or, would you opt out of medical practice altogether, either by retiring or seeking a job that does not entail patient interaction?

These questions take us back to the premise of this chapter, which is that how physicians feel about being physicians is a vital healthcare policy matter. If physicians are largely satisfied with current medical practice conditions and are willing and able to continue in their present role as caregivers, patients and policy makers need not adjust their plans or attitudes.

If, on the other hand, physicians are largely dissatisfied with the medical practice environment and are limiting patient access to their services as a result, or are opting out of patient care altogether, then patients and policy makers must take note.

There inevitably comes a time when each of us requires the services of a physician – be it a primary care doctor or a specialist.

At that point, how physicians feel about being physicians can be the key to both the availability of care and the quality of care we receive.

Are physicians now at the point where they are compelled to limit access to their practices to just certain types of patients? Are they planning to leave the medical field altogether? If so, when the time comes for each of us, will a qualified physician be available to address our needs?

At the Physicians' Foundation, we determined that the best way to answer these questions was to ask physicians themselves, and to do so by conducting one of the largest physician surveys ever completed in the United Stated.

In Chapter Two we discuss what this survey, and the thousands of physician comments it elicited, are all about.

A MATTER OF ACCESS

The information in this book – including the written comments made by physicians – was gathered through the Physicians' Foundation.

A few words are in order regarding who we are. The Physicians Foundation is a not-for-profit organization comprised of physician and non-physician leaders of some 20 state and regional medical societies. Two of the authors of this book are among the group's non-physician executives.

The Physicians' Foundation seeks to advance the work of practicing physicians and to improve the quality of healthcare for all Americans. The Physicians' Foundation pursues its mission through a variety of activities, including grant making and research. Since 2005, we have awarded more than $22 million in multi-year grants to fund a number of studies and initiatives. The Physicians' Foundation was founded in 2003 through settlement of a class action lawsuit between physicians/medical societies and third party payors. Those seeking additional information about the Physicians' Foundation can find it at www.physiciansfoundation.org.

Part of the Physicians Foundation's role is to serve as doctor advocates. Many of our members are physicians and we believe that medicine is a grand and essential profession.

One of our goals is to help ensure that medicine remains a viable endeavor, one that can retain the members it has and attract new, highly capable and motivated young people to the field.

Our concern is that the medical profession itself is under duress and that the healthcare care system is creating conditions that, by eroding physician morale and accessibility, will erode quality of care for all Americans.

Through our physician members we are conscious of the fact that many doctors today struggle with the current medical practice environment, for reasons alluded to in the Chapter One of this book.

The declining state of physician morale is a problem familiar to those who are related to physicians, to those who are friends with physicians, or to those who interact with physicians through work or other venues. Engage a physician in a frank discussion of this subject and many will tell you that the practice of medicine is becoming increasingly problematic.

In the ongoing debate over healthcare delivery, this aspect of the issue – the physicians' perspective – is rarely considered. The Physicians' Foundation's purpose in delving into this matter was not to determine whether physicians are content or discontent with their profession. The purpose was to determine whether how doctors feel about medical practice is likely to affect access to patient services and, by extension, overall quality of care in the United States.

Where have all the doctors gone?

It is important to understand that any move by physicians to reduce patient access to their services or to exit medicine altogether would come at a particularly inopportune time.

The United States today is in the midst of a growing and pervasive physician shortage. Numerous studies and at least one book have been written on this subject, so we will not attempt an in-depth analysis of the subject here.

Suffice it to say that demand for physicians is steadily outpacing supply.

Physician Supply

During the last 25 years, the number of physicians completing training in the U.S. has remained flat at about 24,000 per year. During that time we have added a handful of medical schools, and medical school enrollment is gradually increasing. As referenced in Chapter One, however, to become a practicing physician requires more than four years of medical school. Medical school graduates must complete three or more years of residency training at one of the nation's 800 or so teaching hospitals. While the number of medical school graduates is growing, the number of available residency slots remains virtually fixed.

Year after year, roughly the same number of physicians enter the field. Who these physicians are and how they practice has changed, however. About one quarter of all practicing doctors today are women, and over 50 percent of students entering medical school today are female.

The growing number of women doctors tends to reduce the overall net supply of physicians, since female physicians work approximately 20 percent fewer hours than do male doctors, according to a joint Association of American Medical Colleges and American Medical Association study cited in the June 20, 2009 issue of the *Washington Post*. In addition, there is evidence to suggest that many younger physicians – both male and female

– prefer practices with set hours and regular vacations. In this they are culturally different from the previous generation of doctors, who were accustomed to working back-breaking schedules of 80 hours a week or more.

Net physician man hours therefore are declining at the precise time when demand for physicians is spiking.

Physician Demand

Demand is being driven by several factors, the first of which is simple population growth. Between the years 2000 and 2020, the U.S. Census Bureau projects that 50 million people will be added to the population, through both new births and immigration. That is equivalent to adding the population of England to the U.S. in a just twenty years.

Demand also is being fueled by population aging. The year 2011 will be a landmark, as some 75 million Baby Boomers will begin turning 65, the age of Medicare eligibility. According to the Department of Health and Human Services, people 65 years old or older see a physician at three times the rate of people 35 or younger. When it comes to demographics, Florida is our future. The Census Bureau projects that in 2030 the entire country will be as old on average as Florida, with its many nursing homes and its many doctors, is now.

Technological innovation is a third factor. Each improvement in medical technology creates its own demand. Combine medical innovation with a population committed to living longer and more actively and the burgeoning demand for treatments like Botox, bariatrics and many others is explained.

How Bad?

How bad is the shortage of physicians likely to get?

Projections vary. Richard Cooper, M.D. of the University of Pennsylvania and co-chair of the Council on Physician and Nurse Supply estimates a deficit of 200,000 physicians by the year 2025. The Council on Graduate Medical Education (COGME) projects a less dire but still sobering deficit of over 96,000 physicians by 2020. The Association of American Medical Colleges (AAMC) projects deficits by doctor type as follows:

Projected Shortage of Physicians in 2025 by Specialty Group

Primary care	46,000	(37% deficit)
Surgery	41,000	(33% deficit)
Other patient care	29,000	(23% deficit)
Medical specialties	8,000	(7% deficit)

Source: Association of American Medical Colleges Report, The Complexities of Physician Supply and Demand; Projections Through 2025

In response to these projections, the AAMC has initiated a plan to grow medical school enrollment by 30% by 2015, and recommends that the number of residency training positions be increased by a similar margin.

These numbers don't factor in an important consideration, which is that healthcare reform could expand access to healthcare to millions. During the presidential election, the consulting firm The Lewin Group examined candidate Obama's proposed healthcare reform plan and determined that, if implemented, the plan would cover an additional 26 million Americans and would require an additional 14,500 physicians. The Lewin Group further projected that a healthcare reform plan providing universal access to coverage would require an additional 35,000 physicians.

The Problem in Primary Care

As the AAMC projections above indicate, the brunt of the shortage will be felt in primary care. Shortages will likely be most severe among those doctors who treat the "whole patient" not just an organ or an organ system. Again, these doctors include family physicians, general internal medicine practitioners and pediatricians – the doctors on the front lines of medicine who handle the majority of patient visits generated in the U.S.

Why will there be so few primary care physicians?

The simple answer is that fewer and fewer medical graduates want to be primary care doctors.

A survey printed in the October, 2008 edition of *The Journal of the American Medical Association* indicates that only 2 percent of medical school graduates plan to specialize in internal medicine. In 2006, the American College of Physicians, which is the internal medicine professional society, issued a report stating *"primary care, the backbone of the nation's healthcare system, is at grave risk of collapse."*

The situation is equally bad or worse in family practice. In 2004, the AAFP issued a report stating *primary care will cease to exist in 20 years if changes are not made."* In 2007, 16 percent of residency positions in family practice went unfilled. By comparison, virtually none of the residency positions in orthopedic surgery or otolaryngology went unfilled. Also in 2007, over 50 percent of first year family practice residents were international medical graduates. This is the first time ever that over half of a first year residency class was comprised on non-

U.S. medical graduates, suggesting that family practice is one of those jobs Americans prefer not to do.

Indeed, in the last 10 years, the number of residents choosing primary care has declined by 60%, according to a report cited in the September 12, 2008 edition of *Newsweek*. Reasons for this were alluded to in Chapter One. Primary care physicians are at the bottom of the doctor pay scale, yet still have a very high level of responsibility. As to their lifestyle, it too is relatively unfavorable. Primary care doctors are on call more often than specialists typically are, meaning they must be prepared to see their patients in the hospital at all hours, if need be, even if it means missing baseball games or other family events. Though primary care doctors enjoy a high level of patient rapport, that also is undermined in some cases by third party treatment protocols that limit the autonomy they have to treat patients.

Add it all up and the case for going into primary care is a hard one to make.

Here They Come to Save the Day?

The dearth of primary care doctors is important for many reasons. One of them is that national policy makers are counting on primary care doctors to rescue healthcare from its current cost and quality malaise. Like super heroes, they are being called on to swoop in and save the day.

Though this fact is not always emphasized, healthcare reform as proposed by the Obama Administration, and by many policy makers before it, absolutely depends on the availability of primary care physicians.

It is primary care physicians who are being counted on to reduce costs by providing preventive care, which will catch medical problems on the front end before they become expensive to treat.

It is primary care doctors who are being counted on to coordinate care, particularly for elderly patients, to assure they get the right treatment utilizing the most efficient resources.

It is primary care physicians who are being counted on to collect electronic medical data to determine which treatments work best at the least cost.

None of these goals is attainable, however, without a sufficient number of primary care physicians ready, willing and able to do the job.

Giving Physicians a Voice

But are they ready, willing and able?

We have asserted that the best way to determine this is to ask physicians themselves – to give doctors a voice. Our method was to conduct a national survey – one of the largest surveys of physicians ever attempted.

How the survey was conducted, selected survey results, and questions raised by the survey are discussed in the next chapter.

CHAPTER THREE

TROUBLING QUESTIONS

As anyone who has been to a doctor lately knows, physicians are busy people. Among other things, they fill out more paperwork in a day than many of us do in a month. More than most people, physicians do not have the time or the inclination to complete surveys.

That is why it is remarkable that some 12,000 physicians did so. Not only did they complete a survey of 48 questions, including questions with multiple subsets, over 4,000 physicians supplemented responses to the survey with written comments. Some of these comments, which are featured in this book, are one word exclamations ("Help!"). Others are multiple page dissertations.

We believe the survey offers the clearest insight currently available into the way physicians think and feel about medical practice. It includes over 800,000 data points on specific practice topics as well as insights from physicians themselves.

Here's how the survey was conducted:

Methodology

The Physicians' Foundation selected Merritt Hawkins & Associates, the nation's largest physician search and consulting firm and an AMN Healthcare company, to help develop, disseminate and tabulate the survey.

It was determined that the survey should focus on primary care physicians. Though all types of physicians play an important part in healthcare delivery, primary care physicians are the most frequent point of patient contact. They are the type of physicians most people are familiar with and on whom most people rely for basic care. In addition, primary care physicians are under the most professional duress, for reasons explained in Chapters One and Two of this book. Most important, their services will be relied on to address some of the critical cost and quality of care issues being raised by healthcare reform.

The survey, entitled "The Physicians' Perspective; Medical Practice in 2008" was mailed to 270,000 primary care physicians -- virtually every primary care physician in the country. It also was mailed to some 50,000 specialists. Of the 12,000 responses, approximately 9,000 were from primary care physicians. The survey therefore is particularly relevant to understanding the concerns and challenges facing these types of doctors. Survey results were compiled in October, 2008 and released in November, 2008.

As to the accuracy of the survey, the Physicians' Foundation submitted survey results and methodology to a third party for analysis. Chad Autry, Ph.D., of Texas Christian University, a specialist in statistical analysis, determined that "the overall margin of error for the entire survey is .93% percent, indicating a very low sampling error for a survey of this type (less than 1% error)."

A sobering picture

What did the survey say?

For the most part, it painted a sobering picture of the current state of the medical profession, one that has profound implications for healthcare delivery and reform:

- An overwhelming majority of physicians – 78 percent – believe there is a shortage of primary care physicians in the United States today.
- 49 percent of physicians said that over the next one to three years they plan to reduce the number of patients they see or stop seeing patients entirely, by retiring, working part-time or by seeking non-medical jobs.
- 94 percent said the time they devote to non-clinical paperwork in the last three years has increased, and 63 percent said that the increasing paperwork has caused them to spend less time per patient.
- 76 percent of physicians said they are either at "full capacity" or are "overextended and overwhelmed"
- 78 percent of physicians said that over the past five years the practice of medicine has become "less satisfying"
- 78 percent of physicians said that medicine is either "no longer rewarding" or "less rewarding"
- Only 6 percent of physicians described the professional morale of their colleagues as "positive"
- Only 28 percent of primary care physicians would choose to be primary care doctors if they had their careers to do over. 41 percent would choose a different area of medicine and 27 percent would choose not to be a physician
- 53 percent of physicians have already closed their practices to certain categories of patient

- 34 percent of physicians have closed their practices to Medicaid patients and 12 percent have closed their practices to Medicare patients
- 60 percent of doctors said they would not recommend medicine as a career to young people
- 82 percent of doctors said their practices would be "unsustainable" if proposed cuts to Medicare reimbursement were made.

These selected data points do more than illustrate that many physicians are at odds with the current state of the medical practice environment. As we stated in Chapter One, the purpose of this survey was not to discover to what extend physicians are pleased with or upset by conditions in the medical profession. It was to determine whether or not how physicians think about medicine is affecting access to care and, by extension, quality of care for all patients.

The survey clearly demonstrates that physicians have reached a tipping point when it comes to the practice of medicine, a trend that will significantly affect patient access to their services now and in the near future.

Close to half the physicians surveyed plan to take steps in the next one to three years that will reduce the number or kind of patients they see, or take them out of patient care altogether:

- 11 percent said they plan to retire
- 13 percent said they plan to seek a job in a non-clinical setting (i.e., not seeing patients)
- 20 percent said they will cut back on number of patients seen
- 10 percent said they will work part-time

Many physicians also have closed their practices to certain types of patients, including Medicaid patients, Medicare patients, and patients belonging to certain HMOs and PPOs. They have done so largely because these government agencies and insurers pay them less than their cost of doing business. Sixty-five percent of physicians said that Medicaid reimbursement is less than their cost of providing care, and 36 percent said that Medicare reimbursement is less than their cost of providing care.

Ominously, 82 percent of physicians said that their practices would not be sustainable if Medicare reimbursement to physicians is cut, as has been repeatedly proposed. In such an event, 38 percent of physicians would *stop seeing Medicare patients altogether or reduce the number of Medicare patients they see,* while close to 10 percent would retire.

Questions Raised

These responses raise serious questions about the nature and viability of healthcare delivery and healthcare reform in this country.

Can access to healthcare really be expanded when so many primary care physicians and specialists already indicate they are at full capacity or are overworked and overextended?

Will providing Medicaid and other government benefits to more people actually ensure access to care, when so many physicians already cannot afford to see Medicaid patients?

Can primary care continue to exist as a practice style under current conditions?

Who will provide care to a growing, aging and increasingly health conscious population if doctors walk away from medicine?

The Physicians' Foundation survey raises these and additional questions relevant to both access to care and quality of care in the United States.

We believe the complete survey results merit the consideration of anyone interested in healthcare delivery in this country. Complete results of the survey are included in Chapter Four.

THE PHYSICIANS' PERSPECTIVE: MEDICAL PRACTICE IN 2008

*S*urvey conducted by Merritt Hawkins & Associates, a national
physician search and consulting firm and an AMN Healthcare
company, on behalf of the Physicians' Foundation. Lead author
of this survey and advising consultants for Merritt Hawkins &
Associates were Mark Smith, President; Phillip Miller, Vice President
of Communications, and Kurt Mosley, Vice President of Business
Development. Survey design and layout by Steve Schaumburg,
Director of Marketing and Brand Strategy.

The Physicians' Foundation seeks to advance the work of
practicing physicians and to improve the quality of healthcare
for all Americans. The Physicians' Foundation pursues its mission
through a variety of activities including grant making and research.
Since 2005, the Physicians' Foundation has awarded more
than $22 million in multi-year grants. Additional information
about the Physicians' Foundation is available online at _www.
physiciansfoundation.org_. Principal advisers for the Physicians'
Foundation on this survey were Lou Goodman, Ph.D., President
of the Physicians' Foundation, Walker Ray, M.D., Vice President,
and Tim Norbeck, Executive Director.

Date Conducted

The Physicians' Foundation survey *The Physicians' Perspective, Medical Practice in 2008* was conducted in May, June, and July, 2008

Date Released

Survey results were released in November, 2008.

Surveys Mailed

320,000 surveys were mailed to physicians in all 50 states. 270,000 of the surveys were mailed to primary care physicians, 50,000 were mailed to surgical and diagnostic specialists

Responses

11,950 survey responses were received – a response rate of approximately four percent. Approximately 9,000 responses were received by primary care physicians.

Accuracy Statement

Chad Autry, Ph.D. with the MJ Neeley School of Business at Texas Christian University analyzed survey results and methodology and determined the survey has an error rate of less than one percent.

PART ONE
OPINIONS, PERSPECTIVES AND PRACTICE PLANS

In which state do you practice?

NY	8.47%	LA.	1.43%
CA	8.02%	OK	1.41%
TX	7.79%	OR	1.35%
FL.	5.63%	MN.	1.34%
PA.	4.31%	AL.	1.34%
OH.	4.13%	KS.	0.99%
NJ.	3.66%	NV	0.82%
NC	3.48%	UT	0.79%
MI.	3.35%	AR	0.79%
VA.	3.29%	IA	0.76%
MD.	2.67%	WV.	0.71%
IL	2.60%	NE	0.70%
GA	2.57%	NM.	0.64%
CO	2.37%	ID.	0.61%
AZ	2.24%	DE	0.60%
TN	2.07%	NH.	0.55%
IN.	1.96%	MT.	0.34%
MO.	1.90%	AK	0.34%
WA	1.83%	ND	0.30%
WI	1.72%	WY.	0.20%
MA.	1.72%	VT	0.27%
CT	1.59%	D.C.	0.27%
KY.	1.46%	NH.	0.22%
SC.	1.45%		

What is your medical specialty?

Family practice 27.25%

Internal medicine 20.66%

Pediatrics. 17.50%

Obstetrics/gynecology 13.09%

Other 8.08%

General surgery 5.90%

Urology. 2.11%

Otolaryngology. 2.09%

Orthopedic surgery 1.97%

Cardiology 1.34%

How many years have you been in medical practice (post residency/fellowship?)

26 years or more 25.27%

21-25 years 16.59%

11-15 years 16.03%

16-20 years 15.88%

6-10 years 14.86%

0-5 years 11.37%

What is your gender?

Male 67%

Female. 33%

What is your age?

```
<35 years...............................5.84%
36-40 years ...........................10.94%
41-45 years ...........................13.60%
46-50 .................................17.20%
51-55 .................................21.13%
56-60 .................................12.75%
61-65 ..................................8.36%
65+ ..................................10.17%
```

In what size community do you practice?

```
0-25,000..............................17.90%
25,001-100,000 .......................29.93%
100,001 or more.......................52.17%
```

Over the past five years, the practice of medicine has become:

```
More satisfying .........................5.60%
Less satisfying .........................78.06%
Remained the same .....................16.34%
```

How do you now find the practice of medicine?

```
Very satisfying..........................5.47%
Satisfying...............................28.68%
Less satisfying .........................48.09%
Unsatisfying ...........................17.77%
```

What do you find satisfying about medical practice?

	Most Satisfying	Somewhat Satisfying			Least Satisfying
	1	2	3	4	5
Prestige of medicine	10.83%	24.03%	35.20%	18.57%	11.37%
Financial rewards	3.35%	19.28%	33.70%	20.81%	22.88%
Patient relationships	50.45%	27.72%	15.22%	4.76%	1.86%
Intellectual stimulation	40.77%	40.92%	14.22%	2.87%	1.22%
Professional relationships	18.09%	38.09%	29.40%	10.79%	3.64%
Other	18.35%	18.66%	34.50%	8.23%	20.26%

What do you find unsatisfying about medical practice?

	Most Satisfying	Somewhat Satisfying			Least Satisfying
	1	2	3	4	5
Long hours/no personal time	35.22%	26.75%	21.57%	10.80%	5.67%
Managed care issues	51.60%	25.53%	11.09%	5.16%	6.61%
Malpractice/defensive medicine	49.90%	24.64%	13.69%	5.55%	6.22%
Reimbursement issues	54.24%	25.42%	9.99%	4.35%	6.01%
Medicare/Medicaid regs	45.85%	27.93%	14.78%	5.62%	5.82%
Pressure of running a practice	22.19%	27.69%	27.18%	14.43%	8.52%
Lack of clinical autonomy	20.06%	25.20%	26.95%	17.46%	10.32%
Non clinical paperwork	42.02%	25.79%	30.91%	21.72%	11.91%
Other	22.26%	16.49%	38.42%	10.72%	12.10%

Assess the financial health of your practice

Profitable, but low margins 47.91%

Break even. 22.39%

Healthy and profitable. 17.50%

Unprofitable 12.20%

What do you see as impediments to the delivery of patient care in your practice environment?

	Most Satisfying	Somewhat Satisfying		Least Satisfying	
	1	2	3	4	5
Difficulty w/managed care orgs	39.02%	32.89%	18.55%	6.13%	3.41%
Malpractice/defensive medicine	35.46%	31.47%	21.64%	8.28%	3.15%
Cost of EMR	28.18%	33.46%	24.51%	9.20%	4.65%
Non-clinical paperwork	32.64%	35.04%	23.22%	6.99%	2.10%
Demands of physician time	37.12%	35.46%	20.84%	5.41%	1.17%
Declining reimbursement	62.27%	25.28%	8.55%	2.47%	1.43%
Shortage of PC physicians	19.36%	21.73%	29.19%	17.06%	12.66%

How would you describe the professional morale of physicians you know and with whom you work?

Very low 10.90%

Poor 30.97%

Mixed 52.28%

Positive 5.86%

How would you describe your own professional morale?

Very low 10.36%

Poor 19.85%

Mixed 47.31%

Positive 22.49%

Do you believe there is a shortage of primary care physicians in the United States?

Yes. 78%

No. 22%

In the next one to three years, I plan to:

Close practice to new patients 7.38%
Cut back 20.26%
Continue to practice as I am 51.48%
Seek a non-clinical job within healthcare 13.40%
Retire 10.95%
Work part-time 10.15%
Seek job unrelated to healthcare 10.14%
Work locum tenens 7.54%
Switch to a concierge/boutique practice. 7.04%

If you had the financial means to retire today, would you, or would you maintain your practice for at least a few more years or indefinitely?

Retire 44.95%
Maintain practice 43.42%
Practice indefinitely. 11.64%

If you had your career to do over again, would you:

Choose a surgical/diagnostic specialty 40.96%
Choose primary care 27.34%
Choose not to be a physician. 26.99%
Choose a non-clinical path within medicine 4.70%

If you had your career to do over again, would you: (PRIMARY CARE respondents only)

Choose a surgical/diagnostic specialty 41.03%
Choose primary care 27.69%
Choose not to be a physician. 26.69%
Choose a non-clinical path within medicine 4.69%

Based on what you know today, would you recommend medicine as a career to your children or to other young people?

No. 59.81%
Yes. 40.19%

Which best describes your current attitude to your medical career?

Highly rewarding 22.07%
Less rewarding. 59.29%
No longer rewarding 18.64%

PART TWO
PRACTICE CHARACTERISTICS

Is your practice:

Solo practice 34.18%

Group of 5 or fewer. 26.24%

Group of 6 or more. 21.15%

Hospital-based 9.47%

Other 3.99%

Government 2.98%

Are you employed or are you a practice owner?

Employed 38.44%

Practice owner/partner/associate 61.56%

On average, how many hours do you work a week? Include time spent on clinical, administrative/business, compliance and all other duties related to your practice.

0-20 hours. 3.33%

21-30 hours. 4.07%

31-40 hours. 11.05%

41-50 hours. 18.13%

51-60 hours. 25.36%

61-70 hours. 15.74%

71-80 hours. 12.70%

81-90 hours. 5.11%

91-100 hours. 2.43%

100+ hours 2.10%

Of the total work hours indicated above, on average how many hours a week do you spend on clinical/patient care duties versus administrative/business and other non-clinical "paperwork" duties?

Clinical Patient Hours Per Week

0-10 hours	2.25%
11-20 hours	7.51%
21-30 hours	14.02%
31-40 hours	31.25%
41-50 hours	24.33%
51-60 hours	15.12%
61+ hours	7.53%

Non-Clinical "Paperwork" Hours Per Week

0-10	39.84%
11-20	34.79%
21-30 hours	14.94%
31-40 hours	6.72%
41-50 hours	2.55%
51-60 hours	0.75%
61+ hours	0.41%

In the past three years, has a growing volume of non-clinical duties caused you to spend less time per patient?

Yes	63%
No	37%

In the past three years has the time you allocate to non-clinical duties in your practice:

Decreased 6.11%

Increased 93.89%

On average, how many patients do you see per day? (include both office and hospital-based patients)

0-10 . . . . 7.40%

11-20 . . . . 31.71%

21-30 . . . . 41.28%

31-40 . . . . 13.66%

41-50 . . . . 3.71%

51-60 . . . . 0.99%

61+ 1.23%

Which of the following most accurately describes your current practice?

Full capacity 44.92%

Overextended and overworked 31.37%

Have time to see more patients and assume more duties . . 23.71%

Which best describes your current practice?

Sometimes have time to fully communicate with and treat all patients 50.66%

Usually have time to fully communicate with and treat all patients 36.77%

Do not have time to fully communicate with and treat all patients 12.55%

How would you rate the need for additional primary care physicians in your area?

Moderate need for more primary care physicians......48.67%

No immediate need for more primary care physicians..28.95%

Urgent need for more primary care physicians........21.38%

Are you currently recruiting a physician or physicians to your practice?

Yes....................................65.28%

No....................................34.72%

How difficult is it to recruit physicians to your practice?

Very difficult..........................44.76%

Moderately difficult....................43.82%

Not difficult 11.43%

Have cost/reimbursement or time issues in your practice compelled you to close your practice to any category of patient?

No....................................47.05%

Yes...................................52.95%

If yes, which types?

Practice closed to:

Medicaid patients 33.56%

Some HMO/Managed care patients 30.41%

Certain managed care companies............25.73%

Indigent patients......................16.14%

Medicare patients 11.70%

New patients...........................5.22%

Other 4.13%

Self pay patients 3.99%

Typically, if a patient with an urgent problem contacts your office or is referred to your, how long would that patient wait until the first available appointment with you or your practice?

Same day 70.74%
2-5 days 20.14%
6-10 days 3.60%
11-15 days 2.40%
16-20 days 1.68%
21+ days 1.44%

Typically, if a patient with a non-urgent problem contacts your office or is referred to you, how long would that patient wait until the first available appointment with you or your practice?

Same day 9.92%
2-5 days 38.69%
6-10 days 21.02%
11-30 days 19.29%
31-60 days 6.78%
61-90 days 2.96%
91-120 days 0.80%
121+ days 0.53%

What did overhead run in your practice as a percent of income in 2007?

0-25% 3.48%
26-40% 12.32%
41-50% 21.39%
51-60% 35.77%
61-90% 24.36%
91+% 2.68%

Which, if any, of the following payers provide reimbursement that is less than your cost of providing care? (check all that apply)

Medicaid 64.84%

Some HMO/PPO 43.28%

Medicare 36.10%

CHAMPUS 20.57%

Some indemnity plans 14.14%

SCHIP 13.61%

None of the above 7.35%

Estimate the approximate dollar amount of uncompensated care you provide each year:

0-$5,000 . . . . 6.33%

$5,001-$15,000 . . . . 13.13%

15,001-$25,000 . . . . 15.71%

$25,001 - $35,000 . . . . 11.23%

$35,001 - $50,000 . . . . 13.97%

$50,001+ 39.63%

Describe income in your practice over the last three years

Flat 44.10%

Decreasing 40.14%

Increasing 15.76%

Has flat or declining payer reimbursement affected your practice? (check all that apply)

Unable to provide staff raises 39.86%

Unable to purchase needed equipment 35.65%

Had to reduce charity/uncompensated care 34.62%

Had to reduce time per patient 35.54%

No changes 19.86%

Assume a 10.6% cut in Medicare reimbursement becomes effective October 1, 2008, as has been proposed, and an additional 5% reduction is made in 2009. Under these conditions, which best describes overhead in your practice? (responses do not include pediatricians, who do not see Medicare patients)

If cuts are made my practice would be unsustainable. . . 81.64%

If cuts are made my practice would be sustainable. 18.36%

What changes will you make in your practice if Medicare reduces your fees by 10% or more (responses do not include pediatricians)

Seek new sources of revenue 24.76%

Reduce # of Medicare patients seen 24.48%

Reduce or eliminate charity care 15%

Stop seeing Medicare patients 13.66%

Close practice/retire. 9.29%

Seek a non-clinical position. 8.78%

No changes 4.03%

Do you have the time/money/personnel and/or resources to implement/install electronic medical records (EMR) into your practice? (does not include respondents who already have implemented EMR)

Yes, I have time to install EMR 39%

No, no time to install. 61%

Yes, I have the money to install EMR. 23%

No, I do not have the money to install 77%

Yes, I have the personnel to install EMR. 32%

No, I do not have the personnel to install. 68%

Yes, I have the resources/expertise to install EMR. . . 31%

No, I do not have the resources/expertise to install. . 69%

Which of the following describes your current Emergency Department on-call arrangement?

No on-call duties 48.11%

On call duties, no on-call stipend 43.35%

On-call duties, on-call stipend 8.54%

Are Emergency Department call duties a benefit to your practice or a burden? (includes only those with on-call duties)

Benefit 11%

Burden 89%

Given the alternatives, do you think the United States should adopt a single payer, Canadian style health system?

Yes 42%

No 58%

CONCLUSION

The survey concluded with the following question:

If you could make a statement to policy makers and the public regarding the practice of medicine today from the physicians' perspective, what would you say?

This question was added to provide physicians with a forum for expressing their views on medical practice in their own words. Knowing how busy doctors are, we expected that only a handful would take the time to express their opinions in writing.

Obviously, we were mistaken. Over 4,000 physicians contributed written comments regarding the state of the medical profession – and yes, the great majority of their comments were legible.

What they said is the subject of the next chapter.

CHAPTER FIVE

IN THEIR OWN WORDS

The title of this book is "In Their Own Words," and with this chapter we will focus on what physicians themselves have to say about the practice of medicine in America.

It would take a much larger book than this one to include all the comments we received, so we have selected those comments we felt to be the most representative or those which stated the physicians' perspective with particular insight or passion.

Here is what physicians themselves have to say about medical practice in America, arranged under four thematic headings:

1. AT THE BREAKING POINT

In reviewing the thousands of comments submitted by physicians, several general themes emerged. Many physicians wanted policy makers and the public to know that the pressures of medical practice are coming to a head. For hundreds of doctors who added comments to the survey, the practice of medicine has simply become untenable, for a variety of reasons expressed in the comments below. Statements underscoring the various themes are highlighted in bold.

*"I believe most primary care physicians are **at the breaking point**. There needs to be a grass roots effort to make everyone aware of this."*

~

*"Something has got to be done and urgently to assist physicians, especially primary care physicians, to incentivize medical students to go into primary care and help those of us who are burned out to find renewed joy in seeing patients. Malpractice, government regulations, EMRs, even our own medical associations all have their hands out wanting and expecting more time, money and effort just to maintain what we have. **The whole thing has just spun out of control**. The days of seeing patients as people and establishing relationships are done. I plan to retire early even though I sill love seeing patients. The hassles are just too burdensome."*

~

"My advice to policy makers is to wake up and deal with the primary care crisis before it's too late. When I graduated from medical school in 1983 I would not have believed it if someone told me you can't make a decent living as a primary care physician! Thorough, conscientious internists are a dying breed!"

~

*"I have been in practice for ten years now, the last five years as a private solo practice owner. I'm very disheartened and disappointed over the state of the practice of medicine! The combination of low reimbursement and managed care issues over the last three years has made the practice of medicine almost unbearable. If not for a son who I'm working to put through college and a house mortgage I would quit medicine in a heartbeat! I'm beat, tired and under appreciated. **Sometimes I cry myself to sleep** wondering why I got into all this. Am I paying myself this month? Do I have enough to pay this month's debt and lease?"*

~

"I just want to be able to treat my patients to the best of my ability with all the compassion and excellence they deserve. I want to provide a stable employment environment to my employees without them being overworked on a constant basis. I want to see a profitable practice that grows, expands and becomes successful over time, both financially and in terms of providing excellent care. We need policy makers who understand that they are creating a situation in which these goals will soon be impossible in the United States."

~

*"I am not willing to reduce quality so I see fewer patients per day and my backlog is increasing. I cannot hire new family practice doctors though we are always trying to hire. I cannot continue seeing fewer patients for less money and adding more paperwork requirements. **I've had one nervous breakdown already** and would rather not do that again!"*

~

"I am so mired in this mess that I can't see clearly enough to give any good advice."

~

*"I put everything I have into treating my patients, but it's too much work with too little in return. **I am about to lose my family for nothing.** My children have suffered because of time without their dad."*

~

*"The practice of medicine is an art which has been severely damaged by managed care over the last 20 years. The practice of this ancient art has been 'de-professionalized.' **Physicians are treated like a commodity** – like bedpans or linen – and patients are 'zip-coded' to*

physicians and 'capitated' like a cattle run. Your children and mine are inheriting inferior care and not a healing art."

~

"There are too many regulations, too many middlemen, too much paperwork, too little time to see patients leading to missed or delayed diagnosis, all of which is demoralizing to physicians because we can no longer put patients first. Regulation requirements come first."

~

"I do not see why anyone would go into medicine at this time *and very much regret having chosen medicine as a profession. I would never recommend medicine as a profession to anyone."*

~

"I can't work any harder. My income is 65% in real dollars of my 1977 income, but I work harder and more effectively. I can't recruit new physicians – they'd be crazy to come here. People think I'm wealthy because I'm a doctor, I have no personal life. I could go on and on."

~

"Look around, use your eyes and face reality. Cold blooded robbery is taking place, physicians and patients are being robbed by managed care companies and there is nobody to complain too."

~

"Physicians practice medicine today with one eye on the patient and the other eye on the trial lawyer."

~

*"It has become **almost impossible to care for the poor.** I do, along with my partners, and I make today what I did in 1999."*

~

"Medicine is no longer a calling. It is a losing business opportunity. This is why America's best and brightest no longer chose it as a career."

~

"The system we are currently using is broken. It is held together with band-aids. Why is healthcare, which benefits so many, so regulated when the insurance industry is allowed to financially benefit a small few? It is more difficult to fully immunize a child than almost anything else in medicine. Is that the best we can do?

~

*"Without a radical change **family medicine will experience a painful demise**."*

~

"If I had the chance again I would become a lawyer."

~

"I am frustrated, angry, disgusted and ready to leave medicine all together at this point."

~

"Last year I worked hard, took care of patients in the hospital and office, made referrals, diagnosed and listened to patients. I made $60,000. I paid $20,000 in health insurance since I am self employed and had cancer. Something needs to change."

~

"The insurance companies are getting paid for a 5 star restaurant meal while pediatricians can only provide patients with a peanut butter sandwich, chips and a drink."

~

"There is declining respect and much more suspicion of doctors while at the same time an assumption that doctors must commit no mistakes. This is probably the only field where one is obligated to do one's best and even do work that may have no bearing on patient care and not be reimbursed. A doctor today has no say in what they charge a patient and has no authority to decrease or increase payment depending on the patient's ability to pay."

~

*"Family medicine and medicine in general are at the breaking point, we can not continue to practice in an environment with such declining reimbursement, more demands on our time, and overall personal and professional dissatisfaction. I now make less than 50% of what I made in 2002 and find it difficult to even continue to support myself and my family. It is time to make changes in our healthcare system for physicians and especially for the ultimate benefit of our patients **no matter what we can't take care of patients if our doors are closed**."*

~

"My biggest burden is the amount of student loan debt accrued in becoming a physician. It hinders my plans to grow my practice when $2,000 a month comes off the top of my take home pay."

~

*"We physicians are very tired of being told how to practice medicine by people who never even attended medical school. There are endless rules and regulations that make the entire healthcare system **a bureaucratic nightmare** and only serves the purpose of confusing everyone to the point that insurance companies can deny legitimate claims. Cut out all of the silly rules and middle men and let us practice -- the cost will be cheaper."*

~

"Medicine is more of a headache than it is worth. I get cursed at or disrespected almost weekly by some patient who has no idea about the medical care process. They just want what they want, input and output."

~

"If you cut you're paid more. If you think you're paid less. As a primary care doctor I can see a patient and examine 5 different systems and can care for 90% of their needs in one visit. I am paid less for examining all 5 than each specialist would be paid for each one individually. I expect primary care to be transferred to nurse practitioners, which would be a big mistake."

~

*"People in government expect too much from physicians. We are not a savior of life or health -- all we do is postpone the inevitable and try to optimize health while life remains. **We are not gods, but neither are we slaves**. Americans have become lazy, gluttonous and stupid. They expect medicine to correct all their poor life decisions instead of standing their own feet and using their god-given common sense. Americans need to take responsibility for their own health."*

~

*"I am frustrated by the current state of health care in the U.S. The government has taken the 'profession' out of medicine by micro-managing every aspect. Reimbursements continue to fall while my overhead climbs and **the malpractice climate has become a nightmare!**"*

~

"The practice of medicine has been degraded by the insurance companies, lawyers and the government. We are no longer doctors, we are now health care "providers." Every decision we make is questioned

by insurance companies. *Lawyers see us as 'big pockets.' Patients walk into our office and tell us what they need based on commercials on TV. Are we happy? What do you think?"*

~

"We are being micro-managed by every Tom, Dick and Harry in the United States. *Medicine has become impersonal, businesslike, and full of hassles."*

~

"The cost of running a solo practice and the time needed to manage practice administration are killing me."

~

*"After admitting a patient or seeing him in a consultation, then after following up with rounds at the hospital, after a 12 hour day, you go home. Weeks later you find out you will not be paid for your work. **It is robbery** and does not exist in any other field."*

~

*"I am sure the government does not treat attorneys or other professions this way. I am not sure why we are singled out as a group. **I have lived in this town for 21 years and am going to be done in by Uncle Sam."***

~

"Medicine has become adversarial between doctors, hospitals, insurance companies and patients. It is no longer fixable in my opinion."

~

*"I really wonder what is to become of medicine as a profession? I can barely make a living and it's horribly hard. **Who the heck would do it?"***

~

"We simply are not getting paid for our services such that we can continue. I get less than 60 percent for the same operation as ten years ago, while malpractice insurance is up 300 percent. I can't survive.

~

"I make close to the average American salary of $37,000 though I haven't had a vacation in six years and I'm on call 24/7."

~

*"We are being overpowered by big business, big government and by lawyers. **The little guy who represents the bulk of medicine has no chance for survival.**"*

~

"General surgery is dying. Please help!"

~

"Can you imagine what would happen if your plumber handed you a bill for $60 and you replied, 'I think I'll just pay $32?' In no other profession are services paid for in such an arbitrary fashion."

~

*"Government based health programs such as Medicaid and SCHIP barely cover my overhead. **I plan to quit as soon as I possibly can.**"*

~

*"We have been looking to recruit two physicians for a year now and there has been no interest. I am a busy internist but am paid very poorly ($84,000 before taxes) because that is all that is left after overhead is paid for along with health insurance. **I would never do this again and it is killing both my husband and myself.**"*

~

"Physicians in my community are all in fear of financial collapse. If I continue to practice medicine under this system, I will put my family at risk. I am not willing to do that."

~

"I can't treat patients the way they deserve to be treated because another party now decides what the patient needs even though they do not know the patient. When I first started practicing 24 years ago, I loved medicine. Now it is nothing but hassles from the time I go into work to the time I leave.

~

"As soon as my kids are grown in six years I will become a concierge physician so I don't have to deal with insurance or Medicaid/Medicare. I love being a doctor but I hate non-medical people telling me what to do."

~

*"I see nothing to slow the continuing decline of medicine. Most patients now don't even know what they are missing. **I fear for my grandchildren.**"*

~

"As a recently retired OB/GYN I am sorry to admit that the practice of medicine has deteriorated to a low level. We physicians are held hostage by the insurance companies. It is obvious that physicians lost the battle many years ago and caved into the insurance companies."

~

"Medicine is losing its autonomy, its nobility, its prestige and its respect. Therefore, its pool of bright, qualified, ambitious trainees. Something's got to change."

~

"Medicine is about patients and professional who provide direct patient care. Both are now suffering. The physician/patient relationship has been undermined by lawyers and managed care. Their propaganda has contributed greatly to the loss of the country's soul."

~

"The tangible aspects of medicine such as surgeries or procedures are very well reimbursed. The non-tangible aspects (our knowledge) are not reimbursed well. Managing a diabetic patient for a whole year is reimbursed less than some simple, 15 minute procedure. Primary care physicians are forced to manage the whole patient in 15 minutes or less. This is impossible. We are constantly under pressure to stay longer, see more patients, manage more – and all the while the threat of a law suit lurks. This leads to high burn-out, especially since our pay is decreasing."

~

"For all the education, responsibility and hours we put in what we are reimbursed is a disgrace. **Hairdressers charge more than what we receive for office visits.***"*

~

"The practice of obstetrics is almost suicidal. To pay malpractice would mean I would earn less than the person cleaning my office."

~

"Patients want more from us, we are getting paid less, the cost of practice continues to climb, and we have the constant worry of getting sued."

~

"We are drowning is a sea of regulations and paperwork."

~

"Bean counters have taken over decision making in healthcare."

~

"For two decades, liability, paperwork and frustration from dealing with third party payers have risen. Reimbursement has suffered a slow but persistent erosion. **Many physicians are on the brink of quitting***."*

~

"Reimbursement rates for Medicare/Medicaid/Blue Cross in our county are a sad joke. How can we recruit a physician when they know our county would never be profitable for them? Believe me, plumbers and lawyers wouldn't work for free, and neither should physicians."

~

"I resent that in order to support my family and pay off my student loans I must sacrifice my enjoyment of medicine and see more people in less time. It is not just a disservice to me, but to my patients. I should have become a specialist."

~

"Medicine today is on life support. Imperfect people want perfect results. Despite the preventive measures and education doctors provide, the attitude is 'give me a pill and cure all my ills – but I won't stop smoking, eating or drinking to excess."

~

"Physicians still struggle mightily to take care of their patients but fatigue and discouragement are taking their toll. New docs are jaded and older ones are tired of fighting the battle."

~

"**Doctors are sinking**. We are the ones paying off student loans and overhead while insurance companies are reaping the benefits of our hard labor."

~

"To young college students I would say – don't go into medicine."

~

"Legal regulations, medical liability, insurance costs and insurance company reimbursement abuses are so awful that at age 59 years and four months I retired."

~

"I gave up obstetrics after 23 years out of concern that litigation might evaporate my retirement savings even though I never had a suit decided against me. I work as a clinical instructor to support by GYN practice and do this out of loyalty to my patients and my medical education."

~

"Practicing medicine used to be fun. Now it is a tiring profession. Doctors who treat the whole patient are forced to pack our schedules for less money than last year. We are like everyone – living paycheck to paycheck."

~

"**I regret ever becoming a physician**. This is the only profession in the U.S. with giant conflicts of interest where insurance companies set their fees, my fees and malpractice fees and govern the who, what, how and when patients will receive medical care."

~

"Paperwork! Paperwork is killing us!"

~

*"As a young (33 years old) pediatrician, I feel trapped by my choice to become a physician. Declining reimbursement from payers (especially Medicaid) has forced my employer to cut physician salaries, in some cases by $40,000 annually. This also happened at my prior practice. I have no chance of achieving the income my colleagues were making five to ten years ago. Next year, I will have to see more patients to achieve the same salary I am currently paid. With $100,000 in student loans, I do not know how I will ever achieve financial security. Morale is low in general among physicians in our state. **I would not choose medicine as a career again.**"*

~

"There is still a stereotype of doctors making lost of money and having free time to golf. It's not true. I am the mother of two children ages one to four. My husband and I practice together. He is full-time and I am part-time. We have to see patients every ten minutes to make overhead. Once I get the kids to bed I'm up until 11 pm every night paying bills, employees, taxes, doing CME and finishing the day's paperwork. Patients expect instant access and have no respect for my off duty family time. Unlike lawyers, I can't bill for all the after-hours calls, and patients know they can get free medical care that way – no co-pays. Patients have no respect for our profession any longer, and that's the most disheartening thing."

~

"HELP!"

~

"I have not had a real raise in salary since I started in 1991. I recently became a hospital employee in a probably short-term effort to at least keep income flat. This is not a situation anyone would describe as good for workforce retention. My 'retirement' will likely be an early change in careers."

~

"The current model is not working. Primary care doctors are tired of the continuous pay cuts, reimbursement games, and endless paperwork. As we spend less and less time with our patients because we have to fill out 'prior authorization forms' for every third prescription we write, we become more distanced from the heart of it. There will be a serious healthcare crisis in this country when we walk away."

~

"Prestige and compensation are very far below what they were for physicians in the past and that is already impacting and will ultimately totally change the quality of physicians in terms of intelligence, character, etc. in the future."

~

"As a pediatrician I still enjoy my job seeing patients and talking with patients' parents. But I don't like the fact that right now I'm a medical clerk."

~

"Medicine is not a viable profession anymore. I will retire soon."

~

*"It has become a source of regret and shame that the profession we all whole heartedly accepted to help and alleviate the pain and agony of mankind, has become a monstrous nightmare which is haunting us day and night. We have lost our social status in every aspect and have become robots in the maze of pathways, algorithms, rules and regulations. We are forced to exchange and replace our compassion with robotic rules. **Might as well bring in the robots and computers to deliver healthcare to people.**"*

~

"The joy of medicine has been stolen from physicians."

~

"If I had known 26 years ago that this is what medicine would become, I would have stayed in teaching and never have gone to medical school."

~

"It used to be that physicians were respected and the public assumed the physician was making recommendations out of the best interest of the patient. You could spend time with patients and bill for your services. Now, we need to see as many patients as we can just to cover the cost of the office. Less time with patients discourages physicians from seeing the elderly with multiple problems, all in order to stay afloat. Patients also no longer respect physicians and see us as seeing more patients in order to 'line our pockets' and rushing because 'we don't care.' All the while the amount of information we need to be proficient increases dramatically. **It is impossible to recommend the medical field to anyone.***"*

~

"For primary care to survive, reimbursement must increase."

~

"The only good thing about the practice of medicine is the patients. But I can't afford to see patients anymore. So I'm leaving clinical practice."

~

"It is not worth it anymore. Doctors are treated like service people. The best and the brightest know this and they are no longer going into the medical field."

~

"I enjoy the practice of medicine and my relationship with my patients, but I have yet to draw a paycheck from my practice in the year and a half it has been open. I work as a hospitalist on the weekends but since I've had to put all of the income from that into school loans, mortgages, etc. I'm behind on my taxes. I'm buried in debt and if things don't improve drastically there is no way I can stay in business. There is no way I could be in practice five years or even two whether I want to stay or not."

~

"The debt that we establish while in medical school is difficult to manage for primary care physicians. Increasing costs and decreasing fees have made being a pediatrician a challenge."

~

"It seems we have reached a point where physicians in most specialties have been hit as hard as they can be. I have to pay someone more per hour to clean my house than I have left over treating Medicaid patients for one hour after overhead and taxes! It gets frustrating when it seems that so much of the increasing need for medical care is tied to personal choices such as alcohol abuse, drugs, cigarettes and obesity. My malpractice insurance is at 500% of what it was in 1990 yet my practice gets paid less and less in absolute dollars and even less in real dollars."

~

"Medicine is no longer satisfying for many physicians and many would choose another career path."

~

"Rules, regulations, low pay, malpractice – it is amazing that I still practice medicine. I do so because I love my work. Also, I don't know how to do anything else. I love my work but I hate what medicine has become."

~

"Malpractice has removed the joy of practicing medicine *and the art of practicing medicine."*

~

"Most of us went into medicine to help people. However, we need to survive as well. We made sacrifices, including 12 years of training, enormous student loans, delaying having families, and for what? To be told how, when and how much you'll get for doing your job? I could have done that without spending over $200,000 in student loans!"

~

"Primary care physicians are just plain overworked and underpaid. Medical students are not choosing primary care because they do not see primary care doctors that are happy and the students have decided that medicine will not be their entire life"

~

"Physicians have historically carried the 'burden' of being 'humanitarian' workers. This has led policy makers and the public to disregard the tremendous financial challenges imposed on physicians by managed care contracts which dictate and fix reimbursement fees, increasing malpractice premiums, increasing cost of supplies and the complete disregard of payments for phone services, emergency room call obligations, completion of medical forms and record copies. Coupled with the above are huge student loans for the cost of a medical education and a typical work week of 60 hours or more. Can the policy makers and public honestly view physicians as overcompensated professionals? CEOs, lawyers, accountants, plumbers, electricians, contractors, hairdressers, restaurateurs, retailers and many more professionals have no limitations placed on their income potential by 'governing bodies?' Why should we?"

~

*"The current insurance system is a disaster for OBGYN physicians. Something has to change. **God help us all.**"*

~

"There is no incentive for medical school graduates to go into primary care because (1) no financial reimbursement to counter $100,000 or more in loans, and (2) little prestige. Primary care doctors today are perceived the same as a physician assistant, nurse practitioner and even some RNs. Primary care medicine can be practiced via 'protocols' by mid-level providers, but physicians carry the malpractice liability. What other occupation has built-in pay-cuts the longer one works? Would you tolerate a 40-50% pay-cut over 5-10 years?"

~

*"HELP! If something is not done there will be nothing but nurse practitioners to provide care. **I do not want to grow old in this country!**"*

~

"Medicine is no longer an attractive option for the brightest students. This is the only profession in the U.S. in which the ability to adjust prices to compensate for inflation or increased expenses is absent and controlled by the government. I would never encourage anyone to pursue a career in medicine."

~

"The joy and challenge of medicine is often obscured by the paperwork and fear of litigation despite best efforts. As a young physician, I see myself trying to get out of the field as quickly as possible in order to have a better quality of life."

~

"You win. We're done. Now what? **My advice – don't get sick.***"*

~

"Doctors have become waiters, ready to take orders. Even our own organizations are impotent, or even harmful."

~

"Walk over to your local doctor's office and ask to look at their bills, their schedule, and their waiting room. Then ask if the doctor has time for a cup of coffee. If you find the information staggering with just one pass through, imagine living like that for 20 years."

~

"The myriad rules and regulations we must follow, and the ever present threat of lawsuits that on any day we could make an honest mistake that could cost us our livelihood and even our life savings makes it feel like we are practicing with our hands tied behind our back and a sword over our heads. As for managed care, how would any other hardworking American feel if one day his boss announced, 'I'd like you to keep doing your excellent job, but I'm only going to pay you 40% of your usual salary?'

~

"We physicians are a hard working, overworked, under reimbursed (especially when income is divided into an hourly reimbursement) segment of the workforce. Bright, compassionate future potential doctors are choosing alternate careers due to the inequity between time spent, stress and compensation."

~

"We love our patients. We love our work. But we are struggling to survive."

~

"Pediatrics is totally controlled by insurance companies. They make money while consumers pay more and pediatricians are reimbursed less. Consumers are now choosing to be seen less often because of the cost to them in co-pays. Consumers are being forced to opt for no insurance because of the rising cost of premiums resulting to little or no reimbursement for physicians. The fact is, the insurance companies make money and everyone, consumers, hospitals, and physicians, get financially screwed."

~

"Do not treat us as criminals. The paperwork and barriers to payment assume we are cheats and liars when we are not."

~

"All I can say is I have discouraged my own children from pursuing any jobs or careers in the health field. Enough said."

~

"The low compensation for services has already essentially destroyed the specialty of internal medicine. It is destroying general surgery. It is remarkable that a general surgeon cannot make a satisfactory living by only doing surgery!"

~

"Doctors are the ones on the front lines, sticking their necks out every day in the face of malpractice trying to do good for their patients, and as their reward they get perpetual decreasing reimbursement. And why? Because they don't stand up for themselves. Well, one day, when doctors' backs are pushed way back against the wall, the healthcare system will realize that doctors are kind of important after all, that they do play an important part in society. That perhaps doctors are part of the reason people are living longer and healthier lives. That maybe they do deserve to get paid for what they do."

~

"Trying to practice medicine within the confines of all the various regulators is difficult. We stand face to face with the public who have higher demands because of the information available to them on the TV/Internet explaining not only what may or may not be medically appropriate but also whether or not their desires and my recommendations will be carried out based on what their insurance provider will allow. This not only creates bad public relations but leaves MDs vulnerable to the threat of lawsuits for what it is we might have done."

~

*"In the last 20 years the practice of medicine has lost prestige and is more stressful. In general, physicians are not happy. This unfortunately has changed physician attitudes. **It is difficult to keep smiling when you are constantly being beaten down.** I'm tired."*

~

"It seems the loss of autonomy and prestige of physicians continues every year. Fewer people making decisions in management are trained in medicine. The consequences are more frustration and unhappiness among physicians. This really is the beginning of a crisis that I believe we'll see accelerating every year."

~

"I love medicine – that is why I went to medical school. However, I am losing money on my practice. I continue because I like to see patients, write and lecture. I am using my savings to continue my solo practice."

~

"Doctors are trained to do what they know best – medicine. I think medial practice is starting to plunge downward due to government/

insurance company control. How would you feel if airline passengers started meddling with how pilots fly a plane?"

~

"Only in medicine can you pay one-third of your bill and not get arrested or have a lien placed on your property. The day is coming when physicians will stage a three-day 'holiday' nationwide."

~

"Help me! I want to keep practicing. Please pay me a little for saving lives and curing cancer. I work 28 days a month often at all hours of the night. With no incentive to continue. I haven't had a vacation in five years. I would not recommend medicine to anyone. I regret my fantastic education."

~

"I, for one, am seeking a job outside the USA, *where I'll be paid for my services without having to worry about the huge paper work duties and all the uncompensated care. My job is done here."*

~

"Everyone wants to ride the horse, but no one wants to feed the horse."

~

"I have a huge loan burden. This ruined my finances."

~

"I love my practice. I find what I do to be intellectually rewarding. I love my patients. However, with cuts in reimbursement I have had to take a non-clinical position to supplement my income, and I am still just barely making ends meet."

~

"Practicing medicine has become more and more frustrating. I work more hours today and see more patients and my pay is less than it was 15 years ago. I lose money seeing Medicare patients, but it is hard not to see them. I spend three hours a day calling back patients and doing paperwork, for no reimbursement. Our administration preaches quality, quality, quality, but it takes time to provide quality care and there is no financial incentive to do it."

~

"Policy makers are making medical decisions about things they know very little about. For this they are overpaid and not responsible for any decision they make. Where are they at 3 a.m. when I am called into the ER?"

~

"I work hard everyday but cannot save money for my child. Too much overhead and pay is too low. Even if I take very good care of an OB patient for nine months I only earn $2,000, which does not pay my bill. I would like to quit, but would have to pay money to the insurance company to quit my job. I can't even quit."

~

"Doctors work long, hard hours and are less well compensated than in prior years. The new generation of doctors coming out is more interested in 'working shifts' than focusing on continuity of personalized care. I blame HMOs and the financial pressures. At the end of the day I believe the patients suffer and the big businesses profit."

~

*"I wish my income was 30-50 percent of what the general public thinks I make. I am considered by the big insurance companies to be nothing more than a highly educated blue collar worker without the right to unionize or strike. **I wish our son would have gone into business.**"*

~

"In 1979, liability insurance for a surgeon was $13,000, equivalent to 6 or 7 hernia operations. In 2007, the same insurance is $80,000 and must be paid by performing 120 hernia operations. Reduced resident work hours has had not only a severe compromise of their education and experiencè but resulted in so much cross coverage of patients that errors in medical are rising. The world's greatest patient care and teaching program has been raped."

~

"We are tired, overworked, under paid and over regulated. There are such huge expectations for primary care doctors to know and do everything, yet compensation is so out of whack with what specialists receive. No matter how careful you are, there is a lawyer who is not regulated the way we are who can find someone to find fault with whatever you do. **I should have been an electrician** or gone into business."

~

"Medicine is a broken profession which will never be fixed in my lifetime."

~

"I practice defensive medicine – I probably order unnecessary tests because I feel like the patients expect it, and I am afraid of being sued. I feel burned out and like my

~

which of course I do not, and that puts a lot of pressure on me. And that brings me back to the fear of being sued."

~

"I really like most of my patients and enjoy caring for them but the pain in the neck minority affect my desire to find another line of work. I could make more money going back and being a pharmacist."

~

"As a small business owner and a physician, the price of medical insurance for my employees will eventually drive me out of private practice and into the hospital."

~

*"The only reason I stay in medicine is because I am employed. **If I had to do this via private practice I would work for Safeway.**"*

~

"I spent 20 years in the Army and vastly prefer it to private practice – no problems with insurance approval for procedures and patients could get any tests I ordered or fill any prescription I wrote. Also, my superiors were much less moronic/bureaucratic than my current 'boss,' who is an MBA not an M.D."

~

"The private practice of general internal medicine is suffering 'death from a thousand cuts.'

~

*"**Primary care is in crisis.** My stress, expenses and time have increased yet reimbursement drops. We are having difficulty in getting young physicians here. I feel I made the wrong decision in going into family practice. Many of us feel locked in."*

~

"Diminishing autonomy has made medical practice less rewarding. I wish I had chosen another career."

~

"No time to write, have to see patients! Don't get enough time with my family."

~

"I love what I do! I enjoy my patients. I just don't like paying for that privilege, which is what it is coming to rather quickly for me."

~

"We are in a crisis state. *Most physicians I know would leave medicine now if alternatives were available. This is generally not because of financial reasons, rather the draconian demands of corporate medicine, government demands and insurance company/ corporate issues. This results in loss of autonomy, loss of satisfaction, loss of production, loss of ability to deal with outside stresses."*

~

"Primary care is dead for physicians."

~

"The malpractice crisis and unreasonable patient expectations have sucked the joy out of practicing medicine. We are underpaid and overworked and still expected to be perfect in our judgment."

~

"I may choose to leave medicine because the take-home pay I receive after paying taxes and overhead is not worth the time and effort. If fear for my own ability to receive quality care because of a broken system."

~

"I am currently employed as a physician in a prison. While patient care there is not ideal the inmates get better care than the rural poor."

~

"I went to school for the majority of my life to follow my dream of being a primary care patient centered physician. Since starting practice, I have spent more time and frustration with insurance hassles and paperwork that I would rather spend with patients. Malpractice costs and fears of frivolous lawsuits increase the cost of treatment. I will not live this exhausting life getting up at all hours to care for patients for less than $100,000 a year. I will quit."

~

*"**I have never seen morale so low in the profession.** In my specialty, general surgery, the situation is particularly dire with a decreasing number of surgeons."*

~

"The profession of medicine is still great. The business of medicine is increasingly terrible, especially as we observe other professions (attorneys, investment bankers) doing very well without the responsibility or length of training. I and many of my colleagues believe that medicine has been stolen from us by insurance companies."

~

"Medicine as it is stinks. I did not go into medicine to be told by someone else how to do it for no pay."

~

"In our market economy, what other business can not pass along increases in overhead to the customer? It's like me going to buy a $2 loaf of bread, giving the clerk $1, and saying, 'tough take it or leave it!' This can not continue, or our country will have all foreign doctors in 20 years doing shift work."

~

"Practice of medicine today is slavery."

~

"Primary Care no longer draws the best and brightest because it is not worth it! My 27 year old son has a BS in finance and makes 4 times what I do."

~

"Medicare patients are very time consuming and can not be cared for under current conditions. I consider their care charity and many have a decidedly entitled mentality. **I feel like a slave to a system I that I have no control over.** *"*

~

"Family Practice used to have 25% to 30% overhead and is now at 60% to 70%. Imagine the amount of work that must be produced to dent that discrepancy."

~

"Insurance companies often change the rules and if doctors don't follow the rules they do not get paid for work that has been done. What other business has this problem? Working longer and harder to make ends meet leaves less time for charity work and less appointment time for Medicare and Medicaid patients."

~

"We work our damnedest to provide good care to our patients including charitable care. I provide care regardless of insurance or reimbursement. I deserve to be paid for my work. Legation, reimbursement and insurance issues have tarnished my enthusiasm for continuing to be a Primary Care physician."

~

"Medicine is under valued, under paid and not worth it. I suggest you pick a business career."

~

"MD Primary Care is dead, we are not making them; would never go to med-school in this day and age."

~

"I am now semi-retired, thank goodness I work for the VA and no longer have to deal with the problems of Primary Care practice."

~

"We are getting squeezed to the point that we are becoming miserable. *No doctor that I know is happy. Patients are frustrated by paining high premiums and getting short doctors/patient times."*

~

"A once respected profession has been seriously demeaned and demoralized by allowing cost concerns to override the professional judgment of people who are required to be licensed to serve the public.

~

"As a Primary Care physician in a rural practice I am now in an untenable position. There is no way to see all comers, my practice visits are 70%- 75% Medicare, Medicaid and charity care, and all 3 are under reimbursed."

~

"I don't have time to complete this section!"

~

"The government and insurance companies are practicing medicine without a license. If people want to be doctors they should go to medical school. Medicine is an art it can not be bar-coded, like at Wal-Mart. We are excessively micro-managed, I resent it! ***I was trained to treat patients, not fill out paperwork."***

~

"I left private practice because it was awful. I could not keep up with all of the paperwork, now I work at a student health center. I used to love practicing medicine and my patients loved me, but I could not keep up with the HMO stuff and the Medicare regulations. It was awful and has gotten worse!"

~

"People forgot the time and hours spent before we go into practice – 4 years of medical school and debt and then residency. It is all worth it but we should be financially compensated. The work and time does not bother us but everyone expects to be paid for their time."

~

"Physicians are increasingly loosing control of treatment of their patients. At the same time insurance companies and hospitals are making more. This is not a good time for physicians."

~

"Medicine is a rewarding profession. However, there is too much government regulation, too much paperwork, too many cheatin' weasel lawyers and way too many pencil pushing pecker-heads. Doctors have lost control of our profession. We are letting the animals run the farm. We need to take back our profession from the jackasses!"

~

"My husband and I were in private practice for 28 years and have over $5 million owed to us in uncollectible bills!"

~

"Medicine is no longer enjoyable; it is very stressful and thankless."

~

"I did not become a doctor to run a business. Insurance companies are choking the humanity out of the doctor / patient relationship and their relentless search for profits."

~

"When you include the expense and lost earning years (4 years of college, 4 years of med-school, 3 years of residency) I earn less than if I become a nurse."

~

"I would not do medicine again or recommend it to others."

~

"The practice of medicine was highly rewarding, emotionally, professionally, intellectually, and financially when I began practice. Emotionally it is now draining; enough time can no longer be spent with patients. Reimbursement is no longer enough to adequately pay staff and malpractice has ruined the doctor-patient relationship. These are the reasons the new generation of doctors have lost their compassion and regard medicine as a business."

~

"Primary care is failing due to decreasing reimbursement, rising overhead and increasing paperwork. At my recent medical school reunion those of us in Primary Care agreed that we had been lied to in order to meet the school's goal of producing Primary Care physicians."

~

"I am afraid to even start writing or it will last 20 pages and drive me madder and madder."

~

"Stop! Enough! Why are MDs now valueless? Help,"

~

"The current environment for practicing medicine is not sustainable. Most doctors just want to take good care of their patients. It's getting very hard to do that."

~

"I find the situation in Primary Care to be intolerable. For this I paid off loans for 17 years after medical school?"

~

"Physicians like myself practice in fear of the next malpractice suit that will devastate our practices. We must consistently practice defensive medicine."

~

"Continue to beat us down and I won't be the last physician to quit medicine."

~

"My income has fallen over 70% since 1996. I have borrowed money to stay in practice, I walk in these shoes because these are the only shoes I know and I can not afford to buy or make new ones. I have asked people to walk in my shoes for the last 24 years for a week and so far there have been no takers; however, I still have a job and at least that is positive."

~

"Unfortunately, I do not agree with the direction the USA is going. I am considering leaving the country."

~

"I once loved my field of obstetrics/gynecology. The current healthcare crisis has destroyed this. Low reimbursement, defensive medicine, and outrageous liability have left little for a worthwhile future in medicine. And sadly, as a group of professionals, we are unable to change or control our path."

~

"Medicine has not turned out to be what I thought it would. As a bright young woman who wanted to help and work with people I thought medicine would be a good fit. It is a very stressful job. Worrying about a patient is one thing, and I always take the time to make a thoughtful medical decision. But being awake at night worried because at some point a patient is going to have a poor outcome and I will be sued even if I did everything correctly is not fair."

~

"America's physicians are overworked, underpaid, disenchanted, frustrated, tired, and harassed. Are these the people you want delivering your care?"

~

*"I cannot provide care for $37-$50 per patient when my overhead – malpractice, labor, light bill, rent, and supplies – is $60-$75 per patient. **No one wants to do primary care.**"*

~

"Since moving to a smaller town in a rural, somewhat underserved area, I actually pay to go to work most days. This is primarily due to a high concentration of Medicare and uninsured patients. I have burned through over $100,000 in savings over the past year and will soon have to close my doors or stop seeing Medicare/Medicaid and uninsured patients."

~

"I still believe medical practice is a 'calling' and a respectable profession, but not a secure or desirable lifestyle commensurate with the pressure and sacrifices a doctor makes daily."

~

"Primary care is undervalued, underpaid and extremely vulnerable to liability. **The situation in place now is not sustainable.** *"*

~

"Doctors are burning out, feeling undervalued and very cynical. There is little optimism in the field."

~

"Insurance companies dictate care by refusing to pay for items that do not meet their protocols. They control what, when and how I practice care. It has directly harmed my patients (two this week). Insurance companies need to be stopped. Paying less than overhead is not sustainable."

~

"Please remember that although I love primary care medicine because I love people and relationships, medicine is still my livelihood and my ability to live on my income is becoming very difficult."

~

"In five years I believe private practice will be dead and all physicians will be working as employees."

~

"Today people want a quick and easy and possibly cheap solution to their ailments. They want and demand many services over the phone. They demand we have state of the art equipment, email, websites, electronic medical records, but yet complain of their $20 co-pay. They

do not respect our hours, our sleep. They do not care if we are woken up at 2 am with a slight fever, colic, etc. Malpractice is the pits. We cannot guarantee perfect outcomes. This is biology, not a computer. No one is willing to forgive anymore. I would not discourage anyone from being a physician, we still need them, but if they ask me an honest question they will get an honest answer."

~

"We've been paying student loans for 10 years, and still have 25 years left. We don't fly anywhere or have a gym membership, but even so we are over-drafted on our bank account. The personal sacrifice is tremendous. Our kids get sacrificed the most. We don't have time to take care of our own health. We do a lot of uncompensated work – I'd say 40 percent is free."

~

"I did not go into medicine to get rich. I did so to serve children. I, however, should not have to live paycheck-to-paycheck. The cost of medical education is ridiculous. My loans for school are equivalent to a mortgage. Meanwhile, my salary will never allow me to afford to my own children the opportunity my parents afforded me. ***It's absurd and obscene****."*

~

"To keep the doors open and protect ourselves (malpractice) – do all the paperwork (extra staff) – observe all the regulations (OSHA, HIPAA, etc.) – see enough patients (despite decreasing reimbursement) to pay for all of that…something has to give. Patients are dissatisfied with care. We are constantly told what we can and can't do for a patient by non-clinical people looking at cookbook protocols. Medicine used to be an art – now we are asked to do gold level work with tin as payment. Many procedures cost more in supply costs that we are given

back. I deliver babies because I like what I do but I can't for much longer. I have done the math and in many months we don't get paid after paying for everything else."

~

"After 30 years of rural practice I feel sad about what has happened to physicians. To be paid the same fees I received in 1992?"

~

"When I decided to become a physician at a very young age, my goal was to help people. As I grew older and achieved my goal that did not change, but I always assumed that I would be able to support my family on reasonable compensation for many hours and stress needed to do my job. If I give up the quality of care and personal connection I provide, I could work for a large group and make money. **Or I can continue to be a solo practice doctor and go broke.***"*

~

WHAT ABOUT ACCESS?

Many of the physicians' comments dealt directly or indirectly with the issue of patient access to medical services. The following comments all make some statement regarding how the current medical practice environment is leading to more restricted access to physician time and services.

~

"With the present Medicare requirements for documentation **I spend as much time on documenting a patient visit as I spend with the patient.***"*

~

"When physicians are driven out of business, who will care for the patients? The insurance companies?"

~

"I care for a number of patients without insurance. As a result they turn to the ER, either for primary care or, at the other end of the spectrum, for emergent care that could have been lessened or avoided by access to Primary Care physicians. Further when I do manage their current problem, they have difficulties accessing follow-up care as an outpatient. It is very frustrating to see patients struggling due to lack of insurance and lack of preventive health maintenance."

~

*"The current system of medicine is unsustainable, it is already in crisis. Any further reduction in reimbursement will have dyer consequences **including major physician shortages and substandard medical care.**"*

~

"If regulated too much physicians will either retire early or not work as hard, if paid by the government. Look at Canada, England and New Zealand."

~

*"I came out of medical school $400,000 dollars in debt. I was a single mom while alone in medical school. I went back to school to be a doctor with the intent to treat the poor / Medicaid patients. I was on Medicaid when I was pregnant and was treated horribly. I wanted to get the care I didn't receive to Medicaid patients; however, given the abysmal payment rates of Medicaid and Medicare **soon I will see neither.** I simply can not make my loan payments or save for retirement at these reimbursement rates."*

~

"The health care system in the US is in dryer straights, both physicians and patients are suffering. At the current pace medicine will not be attractive to future physicians. We are heading for a disaster!"

~

"Thank you for surveying doctors. I'm a pediatrician. I was sued 3 years ago and now I have **drastically cut my patient numbers** *and my pay "to pay for the past 9 months" I love my job but the threat of a lawsuit looms over me. I will stop clinical practice in the next year or two."*

~

"I do not understand how our country could make the cost of medical education so high, yet make reimbursement for Primary Care physicians so low. Now everyone wonders why no one wants to be a Primary Care physician!"

~

"I have enjoyed a wonderful career in OB/GYN, I have loved my job and accepted the lifestyle – "patient first, family second." **I gave up obstetrics** *because our legal system has caused the medical system to micro-manage natures process to such an extent that delivering babies is not worth the risk to my health or the sacrifice of my family. I have paid millions of dollars for mal-practice insurance and have never been sued in 25 years. Doctors, nurses, teachers, firefighters and policeman risk their lives and careers daily for little remuneration while athletes play games and make millions of dollars. What a system!*

~

"When we run out of immigrants physicians we will have serious delivery of medical care issues."

~

*"**I have already dropped out of clinical practice.** I planned to retire at age 60 and hope I will never practice in our broken medical system again."*

~

"The practice of medicine today is the worst in history if they cut reimbursement if will encourage doctors to retire early."

~

"I love what I do but can't continue to see my paycheck eroded and still work long hours away from my family."

~

*"Declining reimbursement, high medical malpractice cost and increasing time demands are making the practice of medicine less desirable, leading many of our finer students away from the medical field. This may have long standing implications **regarding access to quality** medical and surgical care throughout the country, especially in rural areas."*

~

"The public demand more and more from their healthcare providers while simultaneously trying to pay them less and less -- that is an unworkable equation. Right now the U.S. fills the gap with foreign medical graduates, but they will eventually become untenable as well. Good luck to those of you who need medical care."

~

*"As with any business, if you continue to decrease reimbursement while costs continue to rise, the business will close. The U.S. is at a point where **the number of physicians may not be enough to care for the population.** Policy makers can not afford to be so short-sided. The damage will take decades to repair and it is already started."*

~

"Pennsylvania is a malpractice crisis state so very few of our graduating residents remain here. Of that very small pool the percentage willing to relocate to rural areas is nearly none similarly specialists are few and far between."

~

*"If Medicare and Medicaid cuts and poor reimbursement continue, **there will be no primary care physicians** able to sustain high quality practices in which to see those patients."*

~

"I can no longer enjoy practicing medicine. I work unbearably long hours, get poor reimbursement and deal with consist frustrations from insurance companies. I can no longer continue to let my job consume my life. I will close my Primary Care / Obstetrical practice at the end of the year and work urgent care."

~

"With looming Medicare cuts a new crisis is pending and many patients will suffer due to poor access to healthcare providers. Ask any Medicare patients in Butler County, OH about their difficulties accessing healthcare providers and they can describe what it will be like for many Medicare beneficiaries soon."

~

*"We are in for a catastrophic event. Less doctors, more under-served areas, more doctors going broke and retiring early and **in the end more difficulty in accessing care."*"*

~

"I teach medical students and they are choosing lifestyle in determining a career, meaning fewer students are choosing difficult disciplines. In 10

years there will be a vast shortage of general surgeons from retirement. They will be retiring at a young age because it's not worth it anymore."

~

"The malpractice situation for ob/gyn is forcing me to stop practicing. I can no longer afford to pay for my malpractice and give excellent care to my patients as I have always done."

~

"I am in solo practice and have watched many of my colleagues retire early. I myself plan to do the same as soon as I am able. I would like to tell policy makers and the public good luck in finding family doctors, internists and geriatricians in another five to ten years. I still like seeing patients in the exam room but as soon as I walk out the door to the piles of paperwork I could just keep walking."

~

*"My practice became unprofitable so **I closed it..**"*

~

"The pediatric clinic at our suburban hospital is closing due to finances and there is no commitment to primary care from the administration. Patients are being transitioned into a federally funded clinic that will undoubtedly deliver sub-standard care."

~

"Pay primary care doctors fairly or soon there will be none."

~

"I am not looking to get rich. I would not have chosen primary care if that was the case; I would like to continue to care for my patients and pay off my medical school debt without going bankrupt. I want to give free or reduced fee care to those with financial need, but if things get any tighter I won't be able too."

~

*"Primary care physicians will **continue to dwindle in number** as long as our reimbursements are so unfairly low. We care for an increasing number of patients with multiple, complex medical illnesses with multiple, complex medications and get very low, unfair compensation."*

~

"Ob/Gyn is being destroyed by the continuing malpractice litigation crisis. With declining reimbursement, $150,000 outlays for insurance is unsustainable. Pregnant woman in the high litigation states will have ever increasing difficulties procuring physician services for their pregnancies."

~

"No MD's will be willing to do primary care. It will be nurses and physician assistants only."

~

*"I am not willing to compromise patient care to see more patients to increase reimbursement. **I see fewer patients and make less."***

~

"I closed my private family practice in 2002 and went to work for the state as a prison doctor. I couldn't even give my practice with 8,000 active charts away. Those patients all had to find new primary care doctors in a community that has few open practices."

~

"I went into Primary Care because I loved the challenge of complex patients and their illnesses. I can not see 30 patients a day and feel that I have given them appropriate care; therefore I've been seeing less each day as well as caring for my hospitalized patients myself. This is difficult financially but at least I can sleep at night."

~

"If primary care is not paid at an appropriate level we will not have enough primary care physicians in the near future. No one will care for Medicare patients."

~

*"I have had a busy, thriving internal medicine practice for nearly twenty-five years. **I had to close my practice** in early May 2008 due to high overhead and ever lowering reimbursements."*

~

"We are in a direr situation. A shortage of primary care physicians will worsen, vastly increasing wait lines."

~

*"Health reform needs to become a priority now or people won't be complaining about the cost in money. Rather they will be complaining about the **cost in lives of loved ones due to lack of accessibility.**. Let's not wait till that extreme."*

~

"Medicare payments must be increased, not decreased, or we will be left with a large, aging, unhealthy population that can not access healthcare except in an emergency."

~

"I am currently employed as a physician in a prison. While patient care there is not ideal the inmates have better access to care than the rural poor."

~

"We are on the brink of a provider revolt, doctors will quite before they take a 10% pay cut, I can happily drive a bus and live in a trailer in Florida!"

~

"Pray, pray, pray a pandemic does not happen in the next 30 years."

~

"The practice of medicine has become a paperwork nightmare. I've about 1 ½ the time available for face to face treatment of my patients then when I started practice 30 years again."

~

***"I will retire ASAP if we have a national health insurance.** Medicare is totally unsatisfactory and has never paid on any claim I submitted therefore I do not accept payment for Medicare, I file the claim and they reimburse the patient and the patient pays me."*

~

"Reimbursement cuts and mal-practice rates have forced me to reevaluate my practice. I stopped providing obstetrical care and delivery 4 years ago. I had many disappointed patients and left a void in our community."

~

"Managed care and the cuts in Medicaid will lead to a severe shortage in Primary Care due to the need to see more patients just to maintain current revenue there will be a drop in patient care and satisfaction and an overall increase in medical cost."

~

"Once driven out of practice by shrinking reimbursement you will not be able to entice me back. I am already making exit plans for the

next 6 – 12 months and will no longer be providing Primary Care to Medicare or managed care patients."

~

"Small office practices will disappear in Primary Care."

~

"Reducing reimbursement will drive doctors out of the profession in droves."

~

"I shall likely seek medical registration in the UK within the next 3 – 8 years, in the event that the US system of delivering medical care continues to devolve as it has."

~

"Unable to continue practicing medicine at this rate, I was one of the few specialist seeing Medical patients and had to stop due to unfair pressures by Medical. I am looking for an alternative source of income to transition away from medicine."

~

"I have closed my medical practice."

~

"It's no secret why there is a shortage of family docs. It's a poorly appreciated, poorly supported occupation. As long as it remains such the frustration will build and the problem will fester."

~

"The next time you need a doctor, call your Congressman."

~

"Soon there will be no one to deliver you grand-children."

~

"We doctors are working harder and getting paid less. Soon there won't be any doctors left to take care of you."

~

"The relatively low reimbursement of Primary Care physicians in comparison with specialist is resulting in an increasing shortage of Primary Care doctors. In the coming years this will have a large negative impact in access to care, disease prevention and overall quality of care in the United States." \

~

"Quality, intelligent young people will no longer go into medicine.

~

"There is an urgent need for more primary care physicians, *they are essential for any health system."*

~

"Health insurance companies put me out of business, they denied everything. I know have a very small specialized practice and work about 10 – 15 hours a week."

~

"I'm in a rural setting and costs are higher because of transportation to get things to me. Patients have to expend more to see me or especially to go see specialist that I have referred them too. Often they simply refuse to go."

~

"There is something wrong with the system when you write-off 40% of your fees. And people wonder why physicians are retiring or getting out of the practice of medicine."

~

"I recently left Primary Care practice and joined a hospitalist inpatient based group due to the extreme hassles of trying to run a private practice. At least 4 – 6 other MD's I know have closed their Primary Care office practices in the last 4 years."

~

*"I'm a 43 year old female physician who is giving up clinical practice in part due to the overwhelming burden of paperwork and micromanaging by insurance companies. Are current delivery system of healthcare is broken beyond repair. **Unless it is fixed, this country will continue to lose 40 something physicians.**"*

~

*"We are dedicated, hard working professionals who have enormous pressures from multiple sources. If this continues **the physician shortage will become much worse.**"*

~

"I have a niece who is extremely bright with straight A's through high school and college. She was considering a career in medicine. Once she analyzed the time and money issues it made no sense to her she followed a different career path where she could earn a better income and have more time. I fear the changes in medicine are making it no longer attractive to the best and brightest, which does not hold well for the future."

~

*"The number of hours, debt needed to receive a medical degree, and stress of being a physician makes me not recommend this field to students. My personal life and time are not fulfilling. **I feel most physicians would retire or quit if medicine is socialized.** Cuts in reimbursement are unfair and many services I have to do are unpaid or underpaid.*

~

"Pennsylvania is a malpractice crisis state and I am in a rural area. Therefore we have had a steady stream of doctors leaving and can not recruit replacements."

~

*"The quality of healthcare is likely to decline as Primary Care **physicians have less time to see more patients** who are more complicated and because insurance companies are interfering in the deliverance of timely appropriate care with drug prior authorizations. Physicians have less time to keep current due to the growing amounts of paperwork. I have recently reduced my patient hours and closed my practice to new patients in order to stay afloat in a 60 hours work week."*

~

"My patients no longer have access to efficient, timely care or the best care I'm able to provide due to my and other physicians' loss of control over our patients' care. Also, my reimbursement has been cut to levels that we have had to eliminate providing many services."

~

"If Primary Care falls, the safety net of the healthcare system falls."

~

"I feel like I provide good service and value for my patients but there is no way I can keep up with demand."

~

*"I practice primarily geriatrics and 50% of the time it does not covering my overhead expenses. If Medicare lowers reimbursement I will have to close my practice **then there will be no doctor in this rural area to care for the elderly.**"*

~

"Medicine is the lowest paying per hour work of any job a smart person with a graduate degree might contemplate, it is unlikely to be able to compete for the best and brightest,

~

"The shortage of physicians is being ignored. *Physicians are being replaced by less educated and trained mid-level. Patients don't realize the danger. Would lawyers or accountants feel that the public would be better served by lawyer assistance or bookkeeper practitioners?"*

~

"By continuing to cut Medicare fees, we are creating a healthcare crisis. ***Soon most competent physicians will have to quit seeing Medicare patients to survive.*** *We need a system of universal healthcare that is privatized and not government run."*

~

"The reason there is a growing Primary Care shortage is that primary care is not valued by insurance companies or by government officials. Leaders say we need a strong primary care base to our healthcare system but never actually do anything about it."

~

"There will be a physician shortage is Medicare cuts are implemented. Also I am familiar with the Canadian and its shortcomings would not be tolerated in the US."

~

"We need more physicians to take care of ever increasing and aging population. We can no longer keep working harder and longer for decreasing compensation. If the current decline in reimbursement

*continues and cost of running a practice increases there will be **severe crisis in access to medical services for all Americans.** "*

~

"While Primary Care should be highly valued as the foundation of our healthcare system it is crumbling. Declining reimbursement for the cognitive work we do combined with increased practice expenses are rapidly putting many of us out of business. Fewer graduates choosing Primary Care while accelerate the lack of access to primary care doctors. We should compensate primary care physicians more equitably for the complex job they do."

~

*"Everyone seems to feel there is no impending crisis but there is. The average age of surgeons, nurses and many other professionals is now in the 50s. Few people are choosing medicine as a career due to declining reimbursement and rising malpractice claims. In 15 to 20 years, **half the surgeons and nurses will be retired and there will be a shortage.** "*

~

"There are certain costs involved with providing the highest quality of care the payors, which ultimately are the people most be prepared to sustain that cost or be prepared for sharp declines in quality. The brightest and best will not continue to choose medicine if other satisfying options are available."

~

*"**Many physician friends are closing their doors and going into another field.** No other field has to pay so much in malpractice cost just to be able to work. It must decrease and soon."*

~

"I closed my practice because I was unable to pay the malpractice rates on the low reimbursement I was paid by Medicare and managed care. I am now retired."

~

"Good luck finding a surgeon who speaks English in twenty years."

~

"Baby boomer demands can not be met in the next twenty years; there is no money for everything that they expect."

~

ELECTRONIC MEDICAL RECORDS

Many policy makers, including members of the Obama Administration, believe that electronic medical records (EMR) are one key to addressing both quality and cost issues in healthcare. How do physicians themselves feel about EMR? A number of physicians who provided comments directly reference EMR. Following are a representative sample of their statements.

~

"EMR implementation will definitely increase overhead and impede productivity. Cost will flow through to physician compensation as all overhead increments do."

~

*"**EMR is a joke** and the greatest risk to patient privacy in existence."*

~

"EMR is not smooth and is not benefiting patient care."

~

"The transition to EMR has been particularly inefficient and not patient friendly. It gets between me and the patient."

~

"The system needs to be fixed from the bottom up; **we need a nationalized electronic medical system** *with embedded clinical decision support systems. We will save loads of money on waste, fraud, administration and we can all be better doctors. With the money saved we can get everyone a basic health care package."*

~

"Electronic medical records increase healthcare cost."

~

"Electronic medical records are not useful if no one looks at them. Paper records can be retrieved on a timely basis with a small invest of time. EMR is not the answer to the health care situation."

~

"The idea that EMR will save money is a joke. *The only money saved occurs because clerical work is now the responsibility of the physician. I hate it, it is time consuming. The amount saved by EMR is almost entirely consumed by payments for computers, support and software. Net saved is zero; with a net increase in physician work hours of 8 – 10 hours a week.*

~

"Implementing an EMR has slowed us down and cut production. The EMR is only as good as the data entered and I am seeing very sloppy data entry by untrained personnel. Supporting education programs for medical personnel and office staff is essential. Who said EMR would eliminate errors? It is scary but the advantages out weigh the problems if done right."

~

"The government and insurance push for EMR is ill-founded. Our office has implemented EMR and it was the worst mistake we have ever made. We can not provide the quality of care we need to provide, we are nearly ruined financially and we spend several hours a day serving the EMR."

~

"The future of solo family practice is dismal. My debt for opening a practice was huge, I can not afford basic cost of living. Never mind EMR, which is still just a dream. Help us!"

~

"EMR is an expensive and non-developed hoax, being perpetrated on naïve physicians and hospitals under the guides of high-tech and improved medical records. With few exceptions the programs are too generic, the scientist are way ahead of the engineers."

~

"EMR technology has not come of age and the current products in many ways are a detriment to patient care. These EMRs needs to be improved before docs are forced to use them."

~

"Quit pushing electronic medical records. The current software is woefully inadequate, waste valuable time and diverts attention from the patients and quality care."

~

"EMR must be a benefit to insurance companies or the government since it most definitely does not improve patient care or benefit the physician."

~

*"EMR is very expensive, **it slows us down but it does provide better medical care.**. We got a grant from the state, the largest given to anyone in the state and the cost of EMR is still prohibitive in time and money. We are going ahead with the grant even though it is a bad financial decision because we think we will be able to provide better medical care to our patients"*

~

"I have almost committed to EMR twice. But they can't decide on a fair amount to charge for my nurse practitioner who helps me a ½ day two to four times a month. I refuse to pay for a full or even a half time license. It is not fair."

~

"Electronic Medical Records will greatly improve what we know as socialized medicine."

~

"I am angry that EMRs are all about billing and not about making my life easier. They all require more physician time. They are not primarily designed for disease management."

~

"EMR is time consuming and a painful startup process taking 15 – 20 extra hours per week for at least 6 months."

~

"The idea of EMR is a good one, but most practices can not afford one. If the government is going to mandate its use then give us a system similar to the VA's EMR."

~

"EMR is a burden, impractical and unnecessary diversion from the main problem our healthcare system faces".

~

"The EMR push is not in the interest of patients, citizens or physicians. It only wastes time, money and directly communicates private health information to the government and creates a very expensive new bureaucracy which is not needed."

~

"A single-payor universal healthcare system based on something like the VA system with it's excellent EMR would drastically increase the efficiency of healthcare in the US by allowing doctors easy access to patient information, vastly improve doctor-to-doctor communication and the ease of using 1 system rather than juggling many systems."

~

*"I have recently moved and have a salaried position and I am part of big group that **already has EMR and it is great!**! Our small group could never have afforded EMR; I think government should help small physician's practices get EMR setup. It makes it so much easier and more efficient to practice medicine.*

~

"Most of colleagues who have implanted EMR have found it costly, time consuming and unsatisfactory. When I receive records form their offices the information is redundant, poorly organized and cumbersome.

~

TREATMENT PLANS

Hundreds of the physicians who provided comments had recommendations for how the healthcare system could be changed.

Many advocate for a single payer system. Many others believe a single payer system would be a grave mistake. The following comments reflect the wide and sometimes contradictory range of opinions physicians provided regarding what should be done to enhance the practice of medicine and improve the quality of healthcare delivery in the United States today.

~

*"A well defined package of healthcare including preventive health care services and mental illness treatment should be **a right and not just a privilege** for all US citizens and should not depend on employment status."*

~

"Odd, isn't it that a nation where people spend billions of dollars on cell phones, Dish T,V the internet, I-Pods, $5 cups of coffee, there is such a push towards socialized medicine. It is not a crisis of finding funding; it is a crisis of individual responsibility, poor decisions and then wanting/ expecting the government (taxpayers) to pick up the tab."

~

"We need a complete overhaul in the current system, doctors spend a lot of years in training and when they go into practice they have a government or insurance company telling them how to practice and how much to charge. When you go to a restaurant do you tell the chef how to prepare the meal and how much you think the meal is worth?, No! Well, doctors shouldn't be in that situation either."

~

"A single-payer plan would be wrong but a simplified system makes more sense. Too much wasted on bureaucracy."

~

"Healthcare should not be beholden to the winds of the free market, corporations and their shareholders. We should not profit off the suffering of human kind, we need universal healthcare."

~

"Managed care and insurance determine the amount of payment, not the doctor. If the huge layer of insurance bureaucracy is reduced it would be beneficial. Patients are paying for bureaucracy whose function is to deny care. High deductible health insurance plans causes a lot of problems, patients get angry when the physician needs to do testing and treatment."

~

"I would emphasize that the practice of "intellectual medicine" is as complex and demanding as that of "procedural medicine" and that this needs to be recognized and reimbursed appropriately."

~

*"We need to switch to a primary care system that is **funded by a "concierge" system**, though not a system just for the rich. Primary care physicians should be given a fairly large sum of money to care for a limited panel of patients with the main focus being keeping patients well and even making them healthier. Quality parameters would be monitored and physician reimbursement would be deducted if quality measures were not being reached."*

~

"Basic healthcare and preventive healthcare should be a right to all USA citizens. Basic and preventive healthcare should be defined and physicians / hospitals should be reimbursed for those services from a single payer system. Expanded healthcare "quality of life healthcare," such as sport physicals, weight management, infertility, etc. should be treated as fee for service by the patient much like cosmetic medicine."

~

*"To increase the number of primary care providers consider **forgiving all medical school debt.**"*

~

"Give the healthcare dollars back to patients. Patients need to assume fiscal responsibility and decisions, choices and cost of healthcare --/ the consequences as well. Get rid of rich and ultra rich insurance CEOs and government auditors that cost money and do not effect quality of care."

~

"Make malpractice insurance optional for physicians. You can not mandate it at the astronomical price of $200,000 per physician! We need huge and significant tort reform ASAP."

~

"Best idea: Do what Taiwan did about 10 years ago! They closely examined and researched the 5 – 10 best systems in the world and designed their own hybrid model to suit their needs. We need to look outside our own borders for ideas first and then design the system, then implement."

~

"Our society must decide if medical care is a right or privilege. If medical care is a right, then the government must provide universal coverage. If medical care is a privilege, then the government and society must acknowledge that it is fair for medical providers to refuse care."

~

"A single-payer system would only make matters worse. I believe more power should be given back to the physician, who is the one practicing medicine and the one who is medically liable if anything goes wrong."

~

"I would tell the public to wake-up and educate yourself, you need to unify and collectively fight back against insurance companies. Politicians and insurance companies are lining their pockets with millions of dollars while you struggle just to qualify for healthcare. It's worse than the Mafia."

~

"We need to follow the lead of European systems. *Do not allow the general public to sit on malpractice juries. Allow people with terminal illnesses to die."*

~

"All the HMO's have been convicted of RICO violations. We don't work for the patients; we work for the insurance companies. Allow us to collectively bargain like farmers who are independent businessmen. We need to form coops."

~

"Patients must be given more responsibility but also more choice when accessing the healthcare system. I have too many patients who come in "just to check their ears before flying" or "just in case" and the insurer gets stuck with the bill. On the other hand, if patients could chose any doctor, even if not in their plan, then the bad doctors (uncommunicative, uncaring, etc.) would be weeded out. Currently in our area patients on low paying plans have very few choices and all end up in one bad practice with poor outcomes. If they could spend their own healthcare dollars they would be better off. High deductible plans with health savings accounts are helping put the decision making back into the hands of patients."

~

"Medical home payments and increased payments for performance can help increase primary care doctors satisfaction."

~

"In the past 18 years of practice the quality of medicine has declined due to pressures of managed care and insurance companies. The autonomy of the physician and the patient / doctor relationship have also suffered. ***Universal healthcare would improve the access and quality of medical care.***"

~

"Rather than the further "industrialization of medicine", increased devotion to patient communications will improve outcomes, compliance and patient / doctor satisfaction with each encounter. Currently US healthcare pays for 'putting out the fire' when patients get ill rather than primary prevention, early diagnosis and treatment. Primary care physicians can take good care of patients and frequently spend more time with no reimbursement. We should not keep putting the cart in front of the horse."

~

"I am or have been a technician and I want to be a physician. Please let me go from technician to physician again."

~

"It is shameful that there are too many patients out there without any form of coverage or insurance. I do not believe in a single-payer system but I believe everyone should have health insurance and I challenge the policy makers to look into universal health coverage."

~

"It would be great to have universal coverage / single-payer for children 0 – 18 years, for full-time college students and for people over 65 years."

~

"We need to innovate new practice models, use mid-levels, have group visits, open access and embrace retail based clinics. How would Michael Dell solve our problems? Not by whining."

~

"We need a federal solution to our medical liability crisis. A good starting point would be to **eliminate private claims against anyone reimbursed through government insurance such as Medicare** *and Medicaid."*

~

"Recognize the role of the physician in the information age is to advise and help patients make informed choices, recognizing risk and benefits associated with those choices and that the ultimate responsibility for personal healthcare and outcomes lies with the patient and his choices about lifestyle and treatment and not on the shoulders of the physician."

~

"The U.S. must find a way to see that physicians only do what they have been trained to do, diagnosis and treat medical problems. The way healthcare is forced to be run is a joke. Why would the country allow expensive, highly trained personnel to fill out paperwork? What a waste of healthcare dollars! We don't need more physicians; we just need to use the ones we have more efficiently. Second, have the American Academy of Family Practice setup and oversee a national billing service that will end insurance denials."

~

"Though a single-payer system seems good for many reasons, I feel it would be run by government bureaucrats who have little or no idea

how their decisions would effect the actual practice of medicine. I just don't trust the government.

~

"I've always believed that government must protect the public and that competent healthcare is a god given right of every human being. We probably should have a competently run government system where every citizen of our country should be provided with this without regards to pre-existing conditions, ability to pay, age, etc. We should be able to provide this type of care for our citizens and if taxes need to be raised then let that be the case. Those who wish to have top of the line care should be wiling to pay out of pocket for private rooms, private nurses and even be able to pick a particular physician for additional charges. Throughout my profession I've come across an assortment of people, including whores, lawyers, insurance sales people and even an occasional politician. I must say the first group has always been the most honest. It is the last 3 groups that will prevent universal healthcare from becoming a reality in my lifetime."

~

*"**The primary need is to return buying power to the patient.** Large deductibles could go a long way towards this with only large bills paid by third parties. There is a need for a government paid system for the poorest 20% of the population."*

~

"Invest health care dollars in direct patient health, not costly regulation, oversight boards, reviewers or computer mandates. These programs detract from bedside and office space services for people."

~

"Please let MDs do what we were trained to do, take care of patients.

~

"Listen to the doctors and the nurses in the trenches. *There is no evidence that pay for performance improves outcomes. Medicare regulations appear to be made very complicated just so they can find some loophole and thus not pay you. The public does not know that medical guidelines are often made by people with a financial interest in the results (i.e., folks with ties to AMGEN making EPO guidelines)."*

~

"Support universal healthcare. Support the medical home. If all patients have access to excellent primary care, it will increase patient and physician satisfaction."

~

"Is it disgraceful that this nation has citizens who can not afford or access healthcare or not afford the treatment they need including meds. We should adopt a single-payer system."

~

"If we have a single-payer system let it be of the quality and availability of those in Congress – air ambulance to Mass General, access to MRI on the weekends, brain biopsies and results in two days, etc. We need reimbursement for non-clinical time, endless forms, pre-authorization, etc, etc."

~

"One of the parts of my job that I find most difficult is having to treat uninsured patients differently than I would if they had insurance, i.e., unable to order needed tests or prescribe medication due to their inability to pay. As a pediatrician it is especially frustrating as my patients are children; however, I am nervous about a government run universal health care system that would

significantly impair my clinical judgment about what treatment course is best for a particular patient."

~

*"Stop frivolous lawsuits and huge settlements. **We are not the enemy.** Decrease the need for such huge malpractice premiums, take care of the elderly and pay decent reimbursement to those of us who care solely for patients in nursing homes."*

~

*"Put a cap on malpractice awards, **yes to tort reform!**"*

~

"I would like to see some changes in Medicaid. Many Medicaid patients abuse the system while those who can't qualify for Medicaid because they work can't afford basic medical coverage."

~

"Government and medicine are a deadly mixture."

~

"Get rid of the large waste caused by coding. The cost of billing personnel coders, my time spent coding is ridiculous and totally wasteful; another billing system that costs less needs to be established."

~

*"Medicare and all government programs are not able to provide all the care people need. **Rationing of care must be done somehow; I would prefer market forces do it.**"*

~

"Single payer isn't the answer, but getting more Americans health insurance is. We're required to have car insurance; we should be required to have health insurance too."

~

"47 million Americans are uninsured but regardless of the patient's health insurance coverage they are entitled to care at the ER. How is the American health care system going to survive giving away free care on a default basis? Universal coverage is a must! See France, which is ranked #1 in the world."

~

"In my opinion the only way to restore any joy to the practice of medicine is to place patients back in charge of their own care by phasing out Medicare and Medicaid and phasing in health savings accounts for all individuals and families. Government might assist with charity care only, healthcare is not a right and it can not be fashioned into one."

~

"Funding for medical training must be completely overhauled. *Medicare funding covers a smaller percentage of trainees each year and has unrealistic criteria. Pay for performance is not patient friendly."*

~

"We need a single-payer system, Kaiser looks like a good model, and we need more medical school openings. There are many qualified students who are turned away each year. Put the emphasis on primary care with an appropriate reimbursement that allows doctors to actually practice medicine."

~

"Let physicians balance bill Medicare patients. Patients need catastrophic healthcare but patients should contract with insurance plans not physicians."

~

"Universal coverage would only further erode medicine unless with it all liability will be placed upon the federal government to effectively indemnify physicians."

~

"Prevention pays for itself in the long term. The obesity epidemic needs to be halted."

~

"A single-payer national health program is absolutely necessary, long overdue and the only rational choice. The major barriers to implementation are pervasive greed and profit seeking from pharmaceutical companies, medical device makers, insurers, hospitals and physicians."

~

"Fine tune medical savings accounts with hybridization (state-assistance and federal income incentives) for less fortunate and/or higher utilizing patients. Greatly cut overhead by doctors and insurance companies by eliminating no value added micro-management. Permit us to recover our profession through the restoration of our autonomy."

~

"I think vaccines should be a government responsibility and should be free to all children nation wide."

~

"While insurance companies continue buying our Senators and Representatives, this situation will get worse. If physicians don't get together and go on strike to show the insurance companies the power of our professional community they will continue under- valuing our work, our skills, our commitment to our patients, and the sense of respect and dedication that our profession demands."

~

"Suggest making consumers bear some cost so that they can price compare. I suggest a 10% of income deductible before insurance or Medicare pays."

~

"It is shameful that this country has so many people without medical coverage. Our system is chaotic and cost would be reduced by a single-payer system."

~

"I believe that returning to using insurance for emergency needs and hospitalization and allowing the rest of medicine to be "pay for service" would be best."

~

"Basic services need to be provided to everyone and catastrophic insurance should be provided to everyone. After that I think that health savings accounts are a way for individuals to choose who they want to see for which services and more judiciously spend their money."

~

"New Zealand and Australia's health systems may be the models to look at."

~

"Physicians should have the right to collective bargain with insurance companies."

~

"Implement incentives for more medical students to choose primary care specialties.

~

"People need to resume some responsibility for their wellness and care that result in injury or disease. People in this country need to decide if healthcare is a priority and be wiling to be sacrifices in other areas to pay for it."

~

"We need a single-payer system; health care should be a right in this rich nation. For- profit HMO's have no place in this business."

~

"Let policy makers be doctors. You cannot swim unless you yourself are in the pool."

~

"We need a British style health system."

~

"The practice of medicine is best when it is a relationship only between a doctor and a patient. Every level of middle men only ruins it further. The government insurers of all kinds are a burden to both patients and physicians and cost health care dollars that should instead go directly to care. If the money spent on healthcare in this country all went directly to care everyone would easily be served."

~

"Medicine is an art, don't make it cookbook medicine. Medicine is a noble profession, just because there a few docs who don't have ethics the majority of docs who want to do well are penalized. Liability is increasing and practicing defensive medicine pushes up practice cost."

~

"Let policy makers have the same insurance as it is available to the common man, let policy makers be paid on a basis of "codes" and not

on salary. Let them be "down-coded" and have money paid lower than their billed amounts."

~

"We need one single-payer that would greatly simplify our over extended, complicated reimbursed health system."

~

"Physicians should be allowed to do what they were trained to do. HMOs and others should stop practicing medicine without a license. Most physicians do what is in the best interest of their patients but they are also human. Like humans in other professions they can make mistakes. Not all bad outcomes in medicine are caused by medical errors.

~

"The rising healthcare cost in the USA is due to the lack of a public health policy / plan. **Establish a public plan to prevent/eliminate obesity**, smoking, drinking, prevent pre-term labor, improve nutrition, exercise and general health. Decrease reimbursement for stroke rehab, end of life / futile care. Malpractice reform, eliminate jurors, have all claims be screened by a community comprised of risk management, physicians, lawyers and ethicists."

~

"It's time to adopt a uniform single-payer system, which may have options for buying additional services for consumers who want more fancy care. People have to take more responsibility for their health and for managing their lives more consciously. **I want to be a "partner" not a "parent" to my patients.**".

~

"We are not a socialistic country and we should not adopt a socialistic form of healthcare. We need less government intervention and need to be paid for what we do."

~

"Develop a two-tiered system – government run medical payer and private insurance payers. Let the market determine fees, services, etc. Stop discounted fee for service. Allow us to refuse care in obviously medically futile cases without retribution. Allow us to practice medicine and not protocols. Free us please!"

~

"Universal healthcare, what are we waiting for? For- profit doctors and pharmaceuticals and hospitals are a shameful injustice. How did we come to this? Milton Friedman?

~

"The medical home concept is the most hopeful idea I've seen in years. *Don't be fooled by someone who promises universal care. This is a fantasy. Improved access and quality are not, but getting all Americans in to a one-size fits all system is unrealistic."*

~

"I am a rural surgeon who sees all comers. I take call everyday. The paper burden and rejections of my billing from all payers and the hoops my people have to go through are unknown in any other profession. Get government out! Go to fee for service, make service charges reasonable and teach American's how to use medical services."

~

"Everyone should have health insurance, similar to social security, paid for by salary deductions."

~

"Do not ruin medical care in the United States by taking more control out of private hands. This power grab of liberals is not American."

~

"Physicians and hospitals should have one fee schedule and should compete on price, this would be the best healthcare plan in a capitalist society.

~

"Practice of medicine is a direct relationship between a patient and his or her physician. I am not a provider! I only treat patients. A physician should treat his patients based on his conscience and faith and should not be dictated what to do by a third party."

~

*"The cost and burden of healthcare on families is overwhelming. It causes many to go without coverage, which is unacceptable in this country. **Universal healthcare is a must!"***

~

"Let us be the doctors and decide proper medical care, not the insurers. Stop treating the insured as statistics and look at them as human beings, unique and individual. Investigate the insurance companies and see where all the real healthcare dollars are going. Educate the public on what's really going on in medicine today.

~

"Reform malpractice legislation, so we don't have to practice 'CYA medicine' and waste money, the patients' and the country's."

~

"Physicians should be incentivized to provide preventive services and disease management services rather than procedural services."

~

*"**Tort reform!** **It works!** I love Texas again. Get rid of insurance companies, use their profits to fund national healthcare. Physicians can run medicine better than insurance executives, Harvard grads, lawyers and politicians."*

~

"While the US medical system is not perfect, it is the best in the world. Nationalizing healthcare would be detrimental to both patients and physicians. Capping malpractice awards and disallowing frivolous lawsuits would help to control medical costs and allow physicians to practice more cost effective medicine."

~

"A single-payer system will not only drastically cut cost but it will improve our economy because businesses will have a lot more to reinvest and new ones can start up. But will our current insurance company / money lobby allow it?

~

*"**A single-payer system will only worsen the existing crisis.** Nothing can be done to prevent the loss of what was the greatest medical system in the world. The rich get richer and the poor get poorer."*

~

"Everyday I am losing money to provide vaccines to my patients. I would gladly accept federal provided vaccines and not charge for anything except administration."

~

"I enjoy being a physician and I'm honored when a patient trusts me to take care of them and their family; however, I am tired of

patients disrespecting my staff. I would like to see patients actually take responsibility for their health and their choices."

~

"Don't punish us for not being perfect – no one is!!"

~

"The best way to fix Medicare and Medicaid is to make them the health insurance plan that all state and federal employees and elected officials have. Then they could experience what is wrong and understand how to fix it."

~

"The government can't run Medicare – how can it handle the entire system?"

~

"Unless major changes occur that reduce healthcare costs, businesses will not be able to provide traditional insurance to employees. Patients will not seek preventive care without insurance and cancer and heart disease will increase, thus costing more to the healthcare system. My income has decreased when inflation is factored for 25 straight years. Reducing physician payment hasn't worked."

~

"I spend 50% of my time on paperwork, a part of practice I do not enjoy. Most of this time is spent proving to insurers that I did my job or dealing with referrals, prior authorizations, proving something is necessary for a patient and battling denials. I could be using this time to see more patients, do more community service. I'm not in the practice of medicine to make it expensive. I do things when I think they are necessary. I don't order tests or medications recklessly, how does some administrator know more about how to care for my

patients than I do? It is time to eliminate all the run-round and get back to good patient care."

~

"I favor a one-payer system; I would rather deal with government regulations than the multitude of regulations and the multitude of insurance companies with their greed and determination to deny care to their subscribers."

~

"I believe in a two-payer system, one public and one private."

~

"I believe a socialized system can work. However, physicians would be salaried and overall probably make less. As such student government loan repayments should be reduced or forgiven entirely."

~

"Many resources are wasted on end of life patients. A tremendous amount of money could be saved by not admitting, ordering tests or over-treating nursing home patients that have no chance for recovery or cure of chronic conditions. Unfortunately, everyone is afraid of lawsuits, physicians profit from treating these patients and families have unrealistic, selfish expectations. Our society wants socialized medicine, but be careful what you wish for. A universal one-payer healthcare system can not work without significant rationing of care. I predict physicians, patients and trial lawyers would be very unhappy with the outcome of such a change."

~

"We now have a 'single-payer' system: it is called Medicare (Single-payer for the elderly). It doesn't work. It pays significantly less to primary care physicians than our overhead, at least in Washington

State. That will make medical practice completely non functional for all but the very wealthy. Lower primary care physician reimbursement means fewer bright, caring young people practicing primary care."

~

"Stop leeching blood from physicians by various parasitic entities at all levels."

~

"Let's get back to healthcare provided by physicians to their patients and not directed by government or insurance companies. Eliminate free standing clinics in pharmacies and freestanding stores and groceries. Instead of patients going everywhere on a whim have them contact their doctor before going somewhere to be seen that never communicates with the physician. Whoever said insurance must pay all of the person's healthcare expenses? Insurance is intended to help not to replace individual responsibility."

~

*"**Leave me alone! I'm a professional**; I don't need 20 unqualified bureaucrats breathing down my neck."*

~

"Limit dollar amounts that insurance companies can spend on advertising. Stop all media pharmacy advertising. Regulate insurance companies. Shift dollars from overpaid specialties to primary care providers. Quality in primary care is directly related to time spent with the patient. Pay primary care physicians for their time."

~

"Decide whether healthcare is a right or a commodity. If it is a commodity continue to allow it to be on the stock market and let pharma companies continue their assault. If it is a right then extend

care for everyone and get a single system with simple rules and we could all be more efficient."

~

"There are millions of children without access to care. There are insured children whose parents overuse the medical system for trivial complaints. Pediatrician visits for illness should have a small patient co-pay to discourage excessive visits."

~

"The U.S. should adopt a single payer system but not a Canadian or English style system. The U.S. should provide Medicare to all of its citizens. Payment for this would not require increased taxes, it would be paid for by using the premium dollars wasted on paying for HMOs and other private insurance companies that siphon off up to 50% of healthcare dollars for non healthcare purposes. Medicare has an overhead of less than 2%. It is not socialized medicine, the doctors are not employed by the government under Medicare, we are self employed. Medicare would be just "an insurance company" more efficient with less hassles run by the government and not by private insurance companies whose primary interest is to supply less healthcare and to increase their own profit."

~

"If you think healthcare is expensive now, wait until it's free!!"

~

"Primary care and specialty care should be a 1 to 1 ratio. Every patient should have a "medical home." Community health centers should immediately receive funding that is doubled. Every citizen should have health coverage and a primary care physician."

~

"In my opinion the most important factor that endangers primary care is the reimbursement disparity that exists between primary care doctors and specialists."

~

"Pilot 'medical home programs' and restore the dignity of primary care physicians."

~

"As the number of physicians remains nearly stable while the U.S. population grows, particularly the elderly, it is time to stop connecting employment with insurance. As insurance companies continue to favor paying for procedure-based specialties, Primary Care physicians feel more like someone with a vocation and have less opportunity to be the diagnosticians we were trained to be. I hate bending over backwards tangling with people whose sole job is to withhold payment from doctors and hospitals."

~

"One can not expect to get Ritz Carlton service at Motel 6 prices."

~

"All the people who have made the rules to provide healthcare should be uninsured for one year and learn how to seek medical care, buy drugs, fill insurance forms and see how it works. Tame the expectations of the population. 100 percent of my patients die; they don't have to be miserable on their way out."

~

"Treat and pay physicians as you would teat attorneys caring for clients needs. If you call an attorney or sent him extra paperwork you would expect to pay him for his time. Why do you expect physicians

to do it for free? Physicians should be running the show in medicine not the government or insurance companies."

~

"Mandate healthcare, especially preventive care, and reimburse prevention for all who live in the U.S.A. Increase funding for more nursing schools and increase scholarships for those who aspire to be healthcare professionals. Decrease the amount of unnecessary paperwork."

~

"I believe that it is fundamentally flawed that many primary care physicians are using hospitalists. I can not begin to list the problems that will arise as the primary care physician is not able to or required to be responsible for the full scope of patient care. I don't think very many people appreciate the unseen cost that will come from this trend."

~

*"I believe the solution is **health savings accounts coupled with high deductible** health insurance. I believe the layers upon layers of non-clinical participants in the system are a burden and they add little if any value to the system. With health savings accounts the market could once again drive the system."*

~

"Do not adopt a single-payer Canadian style health system — and I am Canadian."

~

"Give family doctors compensation comparable to specialists."

~

"Get the insurance companies out of the practice of medicine. Reimbursement should be paid to the patient and not to the

physician. Most of the escalating costs are because of the salaries given to managed care employees."

~

"Have all Senators and Congressmen have a health plan that is not any better than Medicare so they can see how difficult the system is for patients and doctors. Reduce debt to physicians by paying off debt if physicians stay in primary care."

~

"Listen to the primary care and ER physicians. Anything that weakens our primary care system threatens to collapse healthcare as we know it. There will be a huge shortage of primary care as baby boomers retire.

~

"**I don't feel a national health system is the answer.** I am not impressed with the way government runs many of its programs."

~

"We need to spend less on folks in their last few months of life and more on preventive care – blood pressure and sugar control."

~

"I left Canada to get away from a failed socialized healthcare system that did a terrible disservice to Canadian patients. I routinely saw people dying on waiting lists for urgently needed treatment that was rationed due to scarce resources. It is an absolute tragedy which too few people in this country realize."

~

"Almost all physicians are more interested in caring for patients than financial rewards and most physicians are competent and caring.

Those characteristics should be encouraged and the current approach does not do so effectively. Given an opportunity most physicians would negotiate reasonable rates for medical care with patients."

~

"Government has failed at managing health care – look at Medicare. Why does government feel they can expand this to the entire population of the U.S.?"

~

*"To reduce time pressures and third party payer problems **I strongly believe a single party payer is the way**, either run privately or publicly with oversight by physician organizations."*

~

"Australian and New Zealand style health systems merit further examination – but not the Canadian system."

~

"It is well past time for a single-payer system."

~

"Stop beating us up with increasingly fragmented regulations, prior authorization forms and all other machinations designed to reduce patient care time and use up overhead resources."

~

"If the VA medical system or the military medical system is to be the "universal healthcare" that politicians have in mind that would be a grave mistake. I have been to both as a clinician and can confidentially say that the VA and military medical systems are breeding grounds for very bad medicine."

~

"Basic health insurances should be made available to all patients, but those who can afford to pay should not receive free medical care. Without some payment the system would be overwhelmed and access denied to many patients."

~

"Any system which does not emphasize patient accountability for costs will be a disaster. **I believe a single payer system is the worst alternative.** *Health savings accounts with government contributions for those who qualify are the best alternative."*

~

"Stop Medicare and HMOs -- they won't let Medicare patients who need advanced cancer, transplant or other treatments needs be met."

~

"Stop the ridiculous malpractice system in this country. Lawyers advertising at all hours of the day, "will get you the money you deserve and it won't cost you a cent, we won't charge unless we get you the money!"

~

"I suggest policy makers go to an ER and not let anyone know who they are, they will learn a lot by being a patient in a chaotic system. Unfortunately, there is no easy cure for healthcare and universal healthcare would lower the bar even further."

~

"I'm leery of a single-payer system since we live close to the Canadian border. I've heard lots of complaints about it. Maybe we need insurance reform to lower the cost of insurance. CEOs making huge salaries, limits on premiums and eliminating pre-existing condition clauses."

~

"Too much time is wasted by clinical staff jumping through hoops for insurance companies. Our nurses are spending approximately 1/3 of their time on the phone with insurance companies instead of taking time to care for patients. A single-payer system could fix that."

~

"I say no to a Canadian style health system. My family comes from Canada."

~

*"The issue is the increasing burden of malpractice costs and lower reimbursement. I would definitely **bring a class action lawsuit against the managed care industry.** They treat doctors like indentured servants. They also restrict the patient's access to the doctors they most want to see and have to take care of them. The rising costs of medical care are least due to doctors' fees and most due to new technologies such as CT scans, MRIs and other imaging techniques.*

~

*"We have no other option in order to take care of the most fundamental needs of our population. Whatever the cost, administrative burden or powerful lobbying opposition **we must adopt a single payer government insured medical system** for all of our citizens."*

~

"Malpractice decisions should not be made by a jury. There is no way they can appreciate what a true standard of care is. Malpractice decisions should be made by a panel of selected individuals, most with medical experience, from each state. This would put an end to ridiculous lawsuits and would also bring justice to those cases that may be legitimate but can not produce enough contingency fees to attract a trial lawyer."

~

"We need a true universal health coverage plan with options for just private coverage only."

~

"Students must graduate with less debt. *It is financially foolish to pursue medicine as a career when compensation is too little too late. The two areas of life with upwardly spiraling costs are higher education and medicine. The government is responsible for this problem and should get out of both. Government interference is burdensome and cost provocative."*

~

"Competition in the market place for insurance providers would help keep cost of insurance down. I for one would seek alternative employment if we went to a single-payer system."

~

"If we're going to have enough money to take care of everyone (not at a Canadian level but at what US citizens expect) we need to look at the whole system. There is something wrong with a system that 'helps save healthcare dollars' by refusing to give children effective medications while sending insurance executives to conferences in Hawaii. Trying to reduce costs by limiting care to patients, giving physicians less compensation or making more hoops for doctors to jump through is a travesty. I bet drug company CEOs aren't making the same salary they had in 1986."

~

"Universal coverage may be a worthy goal but there are much deeper problems with the healthcare system. Just including everyone in the same dysfunctional system is not going to solve all the problems."

~

"**Allow medical savings accounts** for patients to buy healthcare. Allow high deductible insurance for catastrophic events at low cost by eliminating basic service coverages. Get the government and insurance company interference out of the way and allow patients and physicians to once again decide what is desired and needed."

~

"Let the doctor practice medicine, not just work to comply with never ending regulations."

~

"A national health plan if crafted correctly would allow patients to seek help in a timely fashion and perhaps even engage in health promotion."

~

"The health insurance companies are sucking health care dollars for profit. If all that money and red tape were eliminated we would have enough money to provide excellent health care to all citizens. Please implement a national health care system. If any one wants insurance on top of that they can buy it privately."

~

"I recently became permanently disabled due to multiple health conditions. My dream from the age of 12 was to help women to have healthy babies. I was truly blessed to be able to do this for a time. I wanted to be a physician, not have to worry about paperwork, rules and regulations, accounting, etc. Americans want the best local care for themselves but want to limit it for others. A single-payer system would be very expensive and difficult to accomplish but may be better than the current system, which is broken."

~

"There's an amazingly wasteful duplication of lab procedures and forms that could easily be standardized and streamlined to save time and effort and expense."

~

"Fund Medicare better and quit wasting money on other areas or today's healthcare delivery problems will seem paltry compared to what will develop."

~

"First let me describe my practice. I am a salaried employee of a large state public healthcare system run by a medical school. My patient mix is adults age 16 – 85 with chronic medical diseases. The biggest problem we have is the lack of Primary Care physicians to treat the increasing population. Coupled with this is the huge number of uninsured. It is time to declare universal coverage as a goal to work toward. This does not have to be a single-payer government run system. There are other ways to arrive at this end point."

~

"We need a better system that covers all citizens of the U.S. I found it was hard to get health coverage myself when I was already pregnant – it's considered a pre-existing condition and I had to go on the COBRA plan of my husband's old job. What a mess! If something isn't done soon the system's back will break and we will all be screwed. Only those people working for the health insurance companies will be rich."

~

"Please don't delude the public that universal care will pay for itself. *It is no more likely to pay for itself than the Iraq war could pay for itself."*

~

"Medicine has been hijacked by corporate health systems and insurance companies where money rules and quality of care is reduced to a marketing tool. Those of us who have maintained our autonomy through private practice, honoring the sacredness of the doctor / patient relationship, have done so at great peril. We need to go back to a time where physician offices and hospitals where separate entities and physicians could truly advocate for their patients."

~

"Eliminate the fragmented, capricious, time consuming, bureaucratic, confusing, and wasteful multiple payer healthcare fiasco in the richest country in the world and **adopt a single payer system** *that covers all Americans, young, old healthy and sick. And equitably distribute the healthcare dollar to those providing care instead of making HMOs rich."*

~

CHAPTER SIX

WHO WILL SAVE PRIMARY CARE?

If you have perused this book in even a cursory manner you will have gleaned that something is seriously amiss with the medical profession.

Many doctors are deeply disillusioned with the current medical practice environment. The situation is particularly dire in primary care, where the benefits of being a doctor are reaching a point of rapidly diminishing returns.

Thousands of physicians surveyed by the Physicians' Foundation said they will take steps in the next few years that will reduce the number of patients they see. Thousands of others said they will opt out of patient care altogether, either by retiring or finding a non-clinical position. The majority of those surveyed – 60 percent – said they would not recommend medicine as a career to young people. Many of those who wrote comments reiterated this point.

That many doctors are unhappy with the state of their profession is unfortunate in itself, but much more than the peace of mind and job satisfaction of physicians is at stake. What steps doctors plan to take in their careers and how they intend to practice has a direct effect on quality of care and access to care for all patients. At some point, everyone depends on the availability of physicians, yet access to doctors has become increasingly problematic in recent years, particularly in primary care.

This trend will only accelerate in the event that a national health reform plan is implemented and millions of patients who previously were uninsured obtain some form of coverage. The canary in the coal mine is Massachusetts, which in 2006 passed a health care reform plan allowing hundreds of thousands of the uninsured to obtain medical insurance.

Since then, newspapers have carried headlines such as the following:

> *"Doctor Shortage Hurts a Coverage For All Plan"*
> ~ *Wall Street Journal, July 25, 2007*

> *"Doctor Shortage Looms in Massachusetts"*
> ~ *UPI, July 27, 2007*

> *"In Massachusetts, Universal Coverage Strains Care"*
> ~ *New York Times, April 5, 2008*

Just how long do patients in Massachusetts have to wait before they can schedule an appointment with a physician?

Consider a survey that Merritt, Hawkins & Associates, the physician recruiting firm that conducted the Physicians' Foundation's doctor survey, completed the spring of 2009. This survey examined the time it takes patients to schedule doctor appointments in 15 major metropolitan areas. These cities included:

Atlanta, GA	Los Angeles, CA	New York, NY
Boston, MA	Miami, FL	San Diego, CA
Dallas, TX	Minneapolis, MN	Seattle, WA
Denver, CO	Philadelphia, PA	Washington, D.C.
Detroit, MI	Portland, OR	
Houston, TX		

Like most metropolitan areas, these cities have a higher ratio of physicians per population than other regions of the country. Doctors generally train in big cities, and according to the AMA, 90 percent of physicians practice in urban areas. If accessing a doctor is difficult in these large urban areas, it can be inferred that doctor access is even more difficult in areas that traditionally have fewer physicians per population than the national average – rural areas, in particular.

The city with the longest average wait times to see a doctor, as you may already have deduced, is Boston. Average wait times to schedule a doctor appointment in Boston for the five medical specialties examined in the Merritt Hawkins' survey are as follows:

Average Time To Schedule a Doctor Appointment
Boston, Massachusetts

Specialty	Days
Obstetrics/Gynecology	.70
Family Practice	.63
Dermatology	.54
Orthopedic Surgery	.40
Cardiology	.21

Source: Merritt Hawkins & Associates 2009 Survey of Physician Appointment Wait Times

By contrast, Atlanta, Georgia has the shortest average patient appointment wait times of the cities surveyed, as the numbers below indicate:

Average Time To Schedule a Doctor Appointment
Atlanta, Georgia

Specialty	Days
Obstetrics/Gynecology.	17 days
Family Practice	9 days
Dermatology	15 days
Orthopedic Surgery	10 days
Cardiology.	5 days

Source: Merritt Hawkins & Associates 2009 Survey of Physician Appointment Wait Times

Keep in mind that the ratio of doctors to patients in Massachusetts is higher than any other state, and that the ratio of doctors to patients in Georgia is lower than in all but seven states. The list below shows the ten states with the greatest number of physicians per population (including the District of Columbia) and the ten states with the fewest number of physicians per population.

Physicians Per 100,000 Population

Top Ten	per 100,000
District of Columbia	756
Massachusetts	453
New York.	400
Maryland.	386
Connecticut.	368

Top Ten	per 100,000
Rhode Island	363
Vermont	362
New Jersey	332
Pennsylvania	332
Maine	301

Bottom Ten	per 100,000
Idaho	171
Mississippi	181
Nevada	189
Wyoming	191
Arkansas	203
Oklahoma	204
Utah	208
Georgia	214
Alabama	214
Texas	215

Source: StateMaster.com

The Massachusetts example illustrates that patients in areas with a high number of physicians per population do not necessarily enjoy ready access to doctors, even if most patients have health insurance. What is needed to ensure access is both the right number and kind of physicians, as well as a physician workforce that is willing and able to see all types of patients.

The cracks in the physician workforce, particularly in primary care, already are apparent and will only get worse unless something is done.

But what?

Listen to Dr. Phil

The first step is to embrace the bromide used by Dr. Phil and many other self-help gurus: *"You can't fix a problem until you admit you have one."*

There are still academics and policy makers who cling to the notion that the U.S. has enough physicians -- perhaps even too many. Those who hold this view have long had an influence on government policy and succeeded in the 1990s in persuading Congress to put a cap on federal funds allocated to train physicians. As recently as 2008, the last federal budget submitted by the Bush Administration included cuts to funds for doctor training provided through Medicaid. These cuts were justified based on the premise that the U.S. is training all the doctors it needs.

We must wake up to the fact that this simply is not the case.

We also need to look at the big picture and realize there are no bad guys. Medical specialists, who generally earn higher incomes than primary care physicians, are not the problem. In fact, we need more specialists just as we need more primary care doctors, particularly in areas such as general surgery, urology, oncology and a variety of others. Our rising population, population aging, and advances in medical technology all are driving the need for specialists, just as they are driving the need for primary care physicians.

We need a system in which both types of doctors can thrive.

Rethink Graduate Medical Education

The way physicians are trained in the U.S. follows a somewhat haphazard pattern. All doctors must complete four years of medical school. They then decide what kind of doctors they want to be – family physicians, cardiologists, orthopedic surgeons, etc. Through a computer program they are "matched" with a residency training program, sometimes the one of their choice, but not always. Residency training programs are located at some 800 teaching hospitals located throughout the United States. These teaching hospitals are largely clustered in the Northeast, one reason why Northeastern states generally have the highest number of physicians per population.

Teaching hospitals are subsidized by the federal government for their role in training doctors, mostly through Medicare. They usually have latitude in deciding what types of physicians they are going to train. Teaching hospitals may reduce the number of primary care training slots they offer should few medical graduates express interest in these positions. They also may increase the number of slots in surgical or diagnostic specialties to accommodate growing interest in these specialties.

In short, there is no master plan that determines the overall number and type of physicians trained in the U.S.

The time may have come for a national commission to examine graduate medical education and to more strategically map out a program to ensure we are training a physician workforce that reflects the nation's needs (such a plan was proposed in 1994 by the Physician Payment Review Commission.)

It would be a mistake to dictate to medical students exactly what type of physicians they should be. Personally, we would be reluctant to see a family doctor, a cardiologist or other physician who had selected his or her specialty by compulsion and not by choice. A better idea would be to make it easier and more appealing to become a primary care physician (or other type of physician for which there is a pronounced need). This could be accomplished through providing educational loan forgiveness to certain types of doctors or through other forms of financial assistance. Grants also might be made to establish primary care residency programs on a wider geographic basis, focusing on community health centers or other alternative campuses in traditionally underserved regions. These and similar "carrots" may entice medical students who have an interest in primary care but who are concerned by high debt load and other financial considerations to become primary care doctors.

Bridge the Income and Prestige Gap

Merritt Hawkins & Associates periodically conducts surveys of physicians in addition to the survey they conducted for the Physicians Foundation. In one such survey, they asked primary care physicians a question about where they stand in the medical pecking order (see below):

Relative to surgical and diagnostic specialists, which best describes how primary care physicians stand in the medical hierarchy?

Top Dogs	Equal Partners	Junior Partners	2nd Class Citizens	N/A
0.3%	14.7%	31.4%	52.6%	1%

Source: Merritt Hawkins & Associates 2007 Survey of Primary Care Physicians

As this survey and many of the comments in this book show, primary care has been marginalized and is becoming less and less attractive to medical graduates. Yet, primary care physicians are crucial to both maintaining quality of care and to implementing changes many policy makers are counting on to reduce costs and reform the healthcare system.

Something must be done to improve the status of primary care practice, both in terms of income and prestige.

One model for achieving this goal is the "medical home," which was alluded to in several of the physician comments cited in this book.

The medical home, broadly defined, is a practice model in which a primary care physician, working closely with the patient, leads a team of specialists and other healthcare professionals, who provide for or facilitate all of the patient's needs.

The idea is that all patients (but especially older patients who often have multiple chronic ills) would have a single primary care doctor "quarterbacking" a medical team that will efficiently and appropriately manage their health (with active participation by the patient).

Primary care doctors would be at the center of this system, enhancing their role as the coordinators of care and growing their prestige. Payment systems would acknowledge this expanded role. Primary care doctors would be paid a management fee for leading the medical team, a fee for the services they provide, and additional reimbursement based on the quality of outcomes achieved. The disparity between primary care incomes and those of specialists would lessen.

It's a promising concept, and Medicare currently has engaged a number of medical home demonstration projects which should clarify how well the idea works in practice. Like all proposed healthcare changes, the medical home presents challenges. As the captain of the medical team, primary care doctors in a medical home will have to spend more time with patients, educating them and coordinating their care. Unfortunately, time is something that primary care physicians already have little of. The medical home also assumes that primary care doctors will incorporate electronic medical records (EMR) into their practices, which will be necessary to share information with other doctors and vital to determining which treatments lead to the best outcomes. Even with the money the Obama economic stimulus package allocates for doctors to adopt EMR, it is not a sure bet that they will do so, as some of the comments in this book attest.

Still, the medical home holds promise and it's a start.

Remove the cap

As mentioned above, Congress passed a bill which was signed into law in 1997 that puts a cap on the amount of money the federal government will spend on physician training. Due largely to this cap, the number of physicians trained in the United States each year is fixed at about 24,000.

This cap should be removed and more money should be invested on physician training. The Council on Physician and Nurses Supply, a group of healthcare experts based at the University of Pennsylvania, has called for increasing doctor training by 30 percent, or about 7,000 more doctors a year. The cap on funds for resident training would have to be removed to achieve this goal.

Training a significantly larger number of physicians will require an investment of several billion dollars a year – a large sum of money but only a small fraction of the many billions spent annually by the Department of Health and Human Services, of which Medicare is a part.

Let doctors be doctors

The survey and the physician comments included in this book reflect what many doctors find frustrating about the current medical practice environment. Too much regulation. Too much paperwork.

Too little clinical autonomy. Decreasing time available to see patients and family. Eroding physician/patient relationships.

What can be done to change these things?

This question raises the larger issue of healthcare reform. Many doctors whose comments are cited in this book signaled their readiness to embrace a single payer, Canadian style health system. Forty percent of those surveyed by the Physicians Foundation said that, given the alternatives, they are ready for universal, single payer healthcare. This is probably a significantly higher number than would have responded this way just a few years ago, as most doctors have traditionally opposed the single payer model. However, given the challenges inherent to our current system, many doctors now are willing to throw in the towel and try something different.

On the other hand, 60 percent of doctors surveyed are still opposed to a single payer model, even though they may not be content with the status quo. Some seek a more market based system featuring high deductibles, medical savings accounts and other options to allow physicians and patients to more directly contract with one another for services, as happens in most other professions.

What should be done to reform healthcare is beyond the scope of this book. However, whether we adopt a single payer system, a market driven system, or retain a modified version of the current system, physicians will still be the key providers of care. Whatever system is adopted needs to address this fact and, to as great an extent as possible, allow doctors to be doctors.

This means, first and foremost, reducing the layers of bureaucracy that rob physicians of time needed to treat patients and to stay current with medical trends. One standardized insurance form for all carriers would be a major step in the right direction.

Tort reform is another key to restoring the vitality of the medical practice environment. Physicians should not have to operate under a cloud of fear, knowing that a mistake or a circumstance beyond their control could ruin their reputations and their livelihoods.

Restoring medicine's luster will take creativity and a willingness to try new approaches. A promising idea is a hybrid style of practice pioneered by a group of physicians in Modesto, California and now generally referred to as the "Modesto Model."

In this practice style, primary care physicians contract directly with patients, cutting out insurers altogether. Patients pay a fixed, upfront, annual retainer that insures them both access to and time with their physician. All the time constraints and autonomy issues associated with third party payers are eliminated.

The revenue generated by "retained" patients allows physicians in this type of practice to spend a significant portion of their time -- as much as two days a week -- treating charity or indigent patients. This model has particular appeal because it allows physicians to maintain the patient rapport and clinical autonomy they value while achieving the goal of expanding access to the uninsured and disadvantaged.

Now is the time

We hope that in reading this book you appreciate the reasons why physicians are different from other professionals in terms of their training, responsibilities and the overall environment in which they work.

We also hope that the hundreds of physician comments make clear the ways in which physicians are similar to you and me. They want the latitude to do the job they have been trained for and the opportunity to earn an income commensurate with their value and their skills. These aspirations are important to physicians, but they also are important to anyone who has been or will be a patient.

We have reached a time when an old question merits new consideration:

Is there a doctor in the house?

What we do today will determine how that question ultimately is answered.

BUY A SHARE OF THE FUTURE IN YOUR COMMUNITY

These certificates make great holiday, graduation and birthday gifts that can be personalized with the recipient's name. The cost of one S.H.A.R.E. or one square foot is $54.17. The personalized certificate is suitable for framing and will state the number of shares purchased and the amount of each share, as well as the recipient's name. The home that you participate in "building" will last for many years and will continue to grow in value.

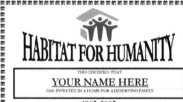

Here is a sample SHARE certificate:

YES, I WOULD LIKE TO HELP!

I support the work that Habitat for Humanity does and I want to be part of the excitement! As a donor, I will receive periodic updates on your construction activities but, more importantly, I know my gift will help a family in our community realize the dream of homeownership. **I would like to SHARE in your efforts against substandard housing in my community!** *(Please print below)*

PLEASE SEND ME _____ SHARES at $54.17 EACH = $ $_____

In Honor Of: _____

Occasion: (Circle One)   HOLIDAY   BIRTHDAY   ANNIVERSARY

      OTHER: _____

Address of Recipient: _____

Gift From: _____ *Donor Address:* _____

Donor Email: _____

I AM ENCLOSING A CHECK FOR $ $_____ PAYABLE TO HABITAT FOR HUMANITY OR PLEASE CHARGE MY VISA OR MASTERCARD *(CIRCLE ONE)*

Card Number _____ Expiration Date: _____

Name as it appears on Credit Card _____ Charge Amount $ _____

Signature _____

Billing Address _____

Telephone # Day _____ Eve _____

PLEASE NOTE: Your contribution is tax-deductible to the fullest extent allowed by law.
Habitat for Humanity • P.O. Box 1443 • Newport News, VA 23601 • 757-596-5553
www.HelpHabitatforHumanity.org

9 781600 377303